YOGA FOR BEGINNERS

(THE BEST GUIDE TO YOGA PRACTICE, CALM YOUR MIND AND IMPROVE YOUR SPIRIT, WITH HEALTH BENEFITS, TRY YOGA POSES FOR FLEXIBILITY, RELAXATION AND STRENGTH)

BY

DENISE FLOW

Copyright 2020 by All rights reserved.

This document is geared towards providing exact and reliable information about the topic and issue covered.

The publication is sold with the idea that the publisher is not required to render accounting, officially permitted or otherwise qualified services. If advice is necessary, legal or professional, a practiced individual in the profession should be ordered From a Declaration of Principles which was accepted and approved equally by a Committee of the American Bar Association and a Committee of Publishers and Associations.

In no way is it legal to reproduce, duplicate, or transmit any part of this document in either electronic means or printed format. Recording of this publication is strictly prohibited, and any storage of this document is not allowed unless with written permission from the publisher. All rights reserved.

The information provided herein is stated to be truthful and consistent, in that any liability, in terms of inattention or otherwise, by any usage or abuse of any policies, processes, or directions contained within is the sole and utter responsibility of the recipient reader.

Under no circumstances will any legal responsibility or blame be held against the publisher for any reparation, damages, or monetary loss due to the information herein, either directly or indirectly.

Respective authors own all copyrights not held by the publisher.

The information herein is offered for informational purposes solely and is universal as so. The presentation of the information is without a contract or any type of guarantee assurance.

The trademarks that are used are without any consent, and the publication of the trademark is without permission or backing by the trademark owner. All trademarks and brands within this book are for clarifying purposes only and are owned by the owners themselves, not affiliated with this document.

INTRODUCTION

Yoga is sometimes described as a Sanskrit, meaning unity. Yoga really means a lot to other people.

Yoga is called Hindu practice, meditation, a life science, a method for enhancing yourself, a path to Heaven, and more.

Many people would say that yoga is more or none of these things.

Was yoga excellent or bad? Yama and Niyama are when you dig at the base of Yoga. Religious rules of ethics and religious observance are not bad.

Nevertheless, someone would eventually say that in Yoga, something terrible exists. Was it wrong to prepare the mind for divine wisdom, creation, and peace?

Yoga is hard to describe.

When yoga is a concept that cannot be specified, the "narrow-minded" one is accused of being a means of weakening religions.

Yoga is going to improve mental, physical, emotional, and spiritual health. It increases the physical and psychological well-being of yoga practitioners. Yoga teaches us a lot.

Through Yama and Niyama, people are told to forgive their enemies, to seek peace, to achieve pureness, to take advantage of the isolation, and to accept self-denial. It should be remembered that any prominent religion holds these fundamental values.

Humanity struggles from minimal thinking. Instead of cherishing cultural diversity, people are too busy debating their differences.

Yoga gives everyone, any faith; an opportunity to see one another is nice. All types of professionals are allowed to enjoy the luxury of retreats and holidays.

If you are an accomplished yogi or new to meditation, there are still the same questions: What is yoga? Why does it work? How does it work?

What is the context of history? Yoga is a long journey that you will experience throughout your life.

Within this post, we offer a short summary of yoga, which ideally draws the attention of those who consider taking a move in the yoga community.

Yoga is widely known for being agile but is much more than physical.

Although the body's benefits are essential (balance, fortification, toning), the inner path takes place when you first placed your foot on the mat.

Yoga (asanas) postures let the practitioner to develop consciousness when entering the present moment. The past and future tribulations records are put aside when you enter the present.

For a traditional yoga class, a brief emphasis is required, and warmup is accompanied by postures that are more active.

Finally, the course concludes with a calming, meditative conclusion that helps you to feel healed and fulfilled.

Yoga is typically practised at workshops or nearby fitness centres. Additionally, there are numerous meditation retreats all around the world for those who want to mix meditation and holidays.

Yoga is everybody's doing. Practitioners of any age, size, and gender will enjoy its benefits. The therapeutic qualities of yoga practice will include pre-existing illnesses, such as cancer, physical disability, and mental illness.

Yoga will help you accomplish your goals, whether you want to lose weight, relieve stress, or enhance your athletic ability.

CHAPTER ONE

What Is Yoga?

A forum was recently held for a group of managers from a conference centre. After some time, the leaders walked the road and met each of them personally. Over a period of time, managers coached each of them. Within an hour for Yoga, the class is structured to balance its personal intent with its professional goals.

We were warned that the HR in charge of this program could not meet expectations since most managers are Yoga practitioners. We nevertheless took the risk as is required and learned what we really assumed to be true. Few people know a great deal about Yoga. We have no prior knowledge with the same thing, though.

We learned the information from different outlets, including news, books, and conversations in the living room. They are mentally capable, but in reality, they are small.

It was a little fun, humorous, not arrogant) because virtually all of them could write a Yoga treatise and it's different functions, types, and advantages, but never had a brief exercise in internalizing it.

They knew the names (especially those of the challenging ones) of some Asanas (sitting and exercise) and Pranayamas (breathing exercises). Clearly, they were very impressed by their knowledge. The practice was meant somehow for people who lived on a different level.

Yoga is considered to be a religion by others, ideology by others, and tradition by some-as in Tantrism.

The government of Malaysia has outlawed yoga, as it is considered a religious tradition that does not adhere to Islamic traditions. Some of this presumption is justified as yoga is stated in Geeta, the religious book of the Hindus, for the first time (to my knowledge).

There is no date for Geeta, and it is not really known when Yoga was performed. Neither faith nor Deity is written by Patanjali himself. It is understood that, like all Indian practices, yoga was passed from the Masters to the pupil in the oral tradition until it was thoroughly described in the Geeta's.

The names of Chapters 2 and 3 of the Geeta are "Yoga of Knowledgement" and "Karma Yoga."

In Chapter II, Stanza 47-60, there is an exhaustive description of "Yoga of Practice" in strokes 61 to 70, "Heart Path" or "Bhakti Yoga" and in strokes 71 and 72, "Renunciation Path" or "Sanyasa Yoga."

After describing in the second chapter the foundations of yoga, the third chapter, "Karma Yoga" honours Arjuna for practice, demonstrating to him that this "course of action" is a way of achieving the end of the "course of understanding."

Inaction or pure renunciation, however, diligent practice and obligation, cannot accomplish Moksha.

Patanjali's only codification of yoga rituals ever appeared in his treatise recognized as "Yoga Sutras." This is the single manual for Yoga Practice for the purpose of this book.

Yeah, as written and explained by Sri Patanjali, the Yoga Sutra is a Yoga Practice Instruction Manual. It is not a religion, nor is it an ideology. This is a step-by-step guide to the aims of yoga. As the human instinct, various schools of thought have interpreted and reinterpreted Sutras in keeping with their purpose.

The Yoga Sutras explain mechanisms and activities through which a natural individual can be so inspired by reuniting with their real source and thereby achieving their maximum capacity through which they live.

The first "Samadhi Pada" defines Yoga's underlying meanings, diagrams, mechanisms, and goals. In 195 sentences (sutras), the whole Yoga Sutra is written-a sutra is just a sentence; simply, a series of words.

Thy name is Brevity Patanjali.
- The first sutra reads in Sanskrit, "Atha Yoganusasanam."
- Atha-Here, now, here, here, here.
- Yoga by the word Yuj, which means joint, united, linked.
- Anusasanam-Training, instructions.
- When he wrote in English, Patanjali would quote, "It is the official instruction of Yoga."

If Yoga means Yuj and Yuj, what is the mix that will be known as Yoga?

This would become apparent once all 195 Sutras are read and merged to appreciate the meaning of several words used, though not clarified, by Sri Patanjali.

The Sutras commentaries are not Sri Patanjali's own. The relationship seems to be that of the body and mind of the Sutra. The binding agent is oxygen.

Therefore, the body, air, and spirit are the three components of Yoga.

We learned the well-known quotations,' Emotion is produced by motion," Physiology is psychology,' which both seem to come from Yuj or Yoga.

The next sutra reads Yogash Chitta-vritti nirodhah, in Sanskrit. Yoga is in English. Chitta is a consciousness field. Vritti-the mind is wandering.

Nirodhah –leaving. Yoga is the truce of a wandering mind to free its restrictive habits from the realm of consciousness.

The primary aim of Yoga is then the mind and ceasing of thoughts that pervert the pure field of consciousness, and the means are corporal exercises and breathing as described in other Sutras.

Meditation is the final target, and asanas and breathing (pranayama) techniques train us for the last.

Therefore, just contemplation is not Yoga, nor is it only asana or pranayama or either while Patanjali says in Sutra19 chapter 1 that certain fortunate people are raised in the state of Yoga and don't have to train or control themselves.

Tada Drastuh Swarupe Avasthanam Tada: Thus, that-termination of thinking is done in such a way.

Sutra: 1.3 in Sanskrit

Drastuh: The button, one in Yoga standing.

In its purest form, in its purest form.
Avasthanam –set up.

Stop thinking cycles is Yoga such that the perceiver is formed in its purest state-the Self in full consciousness.

It prevents the shaping of creation and development so that there is only pure selves-as is. Now that we have a concept of yoga, from the point of view of the Master (Patanjali), we can appreciate both literature and measurable yoga-phenomenon himself.

Any other meaning is tainted as it contains vocabulary that Patanjali did not write himself into the Sutras. Later definitions have done justice not to the originator, but to their own modes of thought.

The author just tried to describe Yoga. The word yoga is sometimes translated as "union" or a corrective system from the Sanskrit expression "yuj." An individual is called a yogi, a woman practicer, a yogi.

The postures/poses. The contemporary western yoga approach is not based on shared values or traditions, but yoga has its origins in Hinduism and Brahmanism.

Yoga has been founded in the southern parts of India by seers or ascetics. The seers studied the natural world and lived as close as possible to the earth, observing the different facets of climate, animals, and themselves.

They were able to cultivate grace, power, and intelligence by studying and emulating the various postures and behaviours of the animal kingdom.

The art of yoga positions has been built through these lives of very disciplined. A set of postures were needed to save the body relaxed and to withstand long stretches of silence in meditation.

Brahmanism stems from the holy scriptures known as the "Vedas."

Such scriptures included instructions and incantations. The fourth book, "Atharva-Veda," includes healing spells and remedies, all of which use medicinal plants. This text gave ordinary citizens the magic and the incantations to use in their daily lives and this

"Veda" tradition can still be found in India's streets today. A further ancient piece of spiritual history, the Bhagavad-Gita, describes itself as a yoga treatise but uses the term Yoga as a metaphysical source.

From this literature, the "eight members of yoga" of Patanjali were created.

Yoga Sutra's principal concern is to
establish the "shape of the spirit," and in the next section, we discuss more this.

The depth.

The Vratyas, who worshipped Rudra, the god of the wind, were a group of fertility priests attempting to mimic the sound of the wind by singing.

They discovered they could create the sound by regulating their breath, and through this breath control practice, "Pranayama" was created.

Pranayama is a breath awareness
exercise in yoga.

The Means.

Upanishads that are the religious teachings of ancient Hinduist tradition have established the road to practice and the way to knowledge into the karma yoga two disciplines.

The pathways were built to allow the student to free himself from pain. The Upanishads ' teaching varied from the Vedas. The Vedas wanted outward sacrifices to the gods to provide a happy and fruitful life.

The Upanishads by Karma Yoga based on the ego's inner struggle to liberate themselves from pain. The sacrificing of the inner self instead of the sacrificing of crops and animals (external) was the central principle, and so yoga was known as the path of renunciation.

Yoga shares some features with Buddhism, which can be traced back to antiquity. Buddhism also emphasized the importance of meditation and avoidance in physical postures during the sixth century B.C.

The first Buddhist to learn Yoga was Siddharta Gautama.

Who is Yoga Sutra, and how did the yoga philosophy evolve?

Yoga Sutra is a set of 195 statements that basically include an ethical roadmap to spiritual life and to the application of the philosophy of yoga.

An Indian guru, nicknamed Patanjali, was considered to be the foundation of classical yoga theory over years ago 2000.

The word sutra simply means "a cord" and is used to denote a particular form of written and oral communication.

The sutras in the student will depend on the guru to translate each philosophy.

The interpretation of each sutra may be adapted to the individual needs of the student.

Yoga Sutra is a yoga system, but it includes no definition of a posture or asana! Patanjali has created a guide to the best future.

The centre of his teachings is the' eightfold path of yoga' or the' eight Patanjali leaders.' There are tips from Patanjali for a happier life through yoga.

Posture and breath control are identified as the third and fourth limbs of Patanjali's eight-strong journey to self-realization in the two fundamental practices of yoga.

Today's progressive yoga is the third exercise of the postures. You can find out all you need to adjust to your lifestyle when you enter a yoga class.

THE EIGHT YOGA LIMBS

1. The Yamas are "morals," with which you live your life: your ethical behaviour:

Nonviolence (ahimsa)–not to harm an object. Integrity and sincerity (Satya)-Not to lie.

Unstoppable (asteya)-Not to rob.

Nonlust — Stop pointless sexual experiences—Romantic restraint and other things.

Non-possession   ornon-grading(aparigraha)–don't hide. Free yourself from gullibility and material wishes.

2. Niyamas (comments).

It is how we view ourselves, our inner discipline: o Purity. Purity is attained through the cultivation of the five Yamas. Treat and look after the body like a shrine.

Satisfaction (santosha). Seek joy with what you've got and do. Take ownership where you are, search for the moment for pleasure and continue to evolve.

Austerity (tapas): Self-discipline growth. Present body, voice, and mental discipline to accomplish a more significant spiritual aim.

Holy text research (svadhyaya). Training and study books that inspire you and educate you.

Live in the Divine mind (Ishvara-pranidhana). Be devoted to something that is your creator, or anything that you consider as being sacred.

3. Asana (postures). Asana.

These are the poses in yoga: o To build a relaxed body, to sit and simply feel for a long time. You will still control your thoughts because you can manage your organization. Asana was used by Patanjali and other old yogis to train the body for meditation.

Even the repetition of yoga positions can improve one's wellbeing. This can begin at any age and any moment.

When we get older, do you remember the last time you sit down to pick up something and how you felt? Think that you are aged in the '50s, '60s, 70, so you can always move your toes or sit on one hip. Are you conscious that the bulk of elderly accidents are caused by falls? We appear to lose our equilibrium when we grow older and do something that definitely helps.

The hand fourth, breath awareness, is a reliable tool to use anytime you choose to practice yoga and relaxation.

4. Pranayama (breathing)–Breathing control: inhalation, air holding, and exhalation o Relaxation and meditation are better done by breathing. Prana is the life force of each of us by our breath. Prana is the energy that resides everywhere.

5. Pratyahara (sense withdrawal).

Pratyahara is the removal of a sense. This occurs during sleep, relaxation, or yoga pose exercise. You can focus and concentrate and not be overwhelmed by external sights as you practice Pratyahara.

6. Dharana (concentration), instruct the mind to focus.

There is no sense of time when focusing. The goal is to hold the
mind on one subject, for example, and to remove away thoughts. Real Dharana is when the brain can comfortably focus.

7. Dhyani (meditation), meditation status.

Concentration (Dharana) contributes to meditation status. In contemplation, you have an enhanced sense of consciousness, and you become one with the world. It's not worthy of disruptions.

8. Samadhi (absorption),-happiness.

Absolute happiness is meditation's ultimate goal. It is a state of unity with yourself and with the creator of the divine, as you and the earth become one.

The eight limbs all function together: the top five include the body and brain, the niyama asana, the pranayama, and the pratyahara.

They are the foundation of yoga and offer a forum for spiritual life. The last three contribute to healing the spirit. They were built to help the practitioner attain spiritual maturity or unification.

WHY DO YOU PICK THE BEST KIND OF YOGA FOR YOU?

The style of yoga that you select is a person's choice, and so why we look here to help you off. Many forms keep the positions longer, and others shift quicker. Some types focus on body balance, and others vary in pacing and use of postures, reflection, and spiritual awareness. All are adaptable to the physical condition of the pupil.

You will then assess your psychological and physical needs in what Yoga form. You may just want to exercise regularly, concentrate on improving your versatility or equilibrium. Would you want to focus more on sleep or the wellness aspects? Many schools teach calm, and some rely on resilience and endurance.

Check a couple of different classes in your city. Also, within teachers of a similar style, the way the student likes the lesson will be different. It is essential to choose an instructor that you feel confident with so that you can really enjoy and thereby build longevity.

Once you continue to understand the positions and adjust them for your body, you should also feel confident practising at home! Both forms of yoga include patterns that function in multiple areas of the body.

You can continue the day with a fifteen-minute session in the morning. With little time and experience, the body will feel dense and bright, and there is an option for you to create your routines.

The Major Systems of Yoga Hatha and Yoga Raja Yoga are the two primary forms of yoga. Yoga Raja is depended on Patanjali's Yoga Eight Limbs in the Sutras Yoga. Yoga Raja is among of Hindu philosophy's traditional Indian system.

Hatha Yoga is also a specific form of yoga created by Swatmarama, a 15th century yogic sage in India. The "Hatha Yoga Pradipika" was compiled by Swatmarama, who implemented the Hatha Yoga system.

Hatha Yoga comes from a number of practices. It comes from the Buddhist scriptures, including the Hinayana (straight path) and the Mahayana (straight path). It is also focused on the Tantra traditions, including Vajrayana (sexuality issues) and Sahajayana (the natural way).

There are various types or forms of the yoga of Hatha Yoga. The method of yoga incorporates postures, breathing techniques, and calming activities to work in the physical space of the body.

Swatmarama's Hatha Yoga is distinct from Patanjali's Raja Yoga in that it emphasizes on Shatkarma, "purification of the body," as a means of "purifying the mind" and "working life." Patanjali starts with the "cleanness of soul and mind," and then with postures and breathing, "the body."

The Major Yoga Schools Around forty-four leading schools of yoga and many others say to be yogic.

Two of the primary schools are Raja Yoga and Hatha Yoga. Pranayama Yoga and Kundalini Yoga are both available from Hatha. From Raja are Jnana, Karma, Bhakti, Astanga, and Iyengar.

Hatha-born Yoga types include pranayama yoga. The term pranayama means prana, energy, and Ayama. The action of pranayama yoga is defined as breath control, prolongation, extension, duration, stretch, and power. Some pranayama breath exercises are used in general Hatha Yoga (to correct breathing problems).

This school of yoga is based solely on Prana (energy of life). There are about 99 different postures, all of which are based on repetitive movement or equivalent.

Pranayama also refers to Spiritual force or the force of the entire universe, which manifests itself through the phenomenon of breathing as a conscious being in us.

The practice of Yogi Bhajan, who took the form to the west in 1969, is Kundalini Yoga.

This is a strongly mystical approach to hatha yoga that includes singing, meditation, and airing exercises, both of which are used to enhance the kundalini strength at the base of the spine.

Raja Yoga forms include Raja Yoga / Ashtanga Yoga Raja, royal or royal. It is focused on guiding the power of one's life to control the mind and emotions. And the emphasis should be on the topic of contemplation, namely the Devine.

Ashtanga Yoga or Raja Yoga is one of Hinduism's four main yogic routes.

Ashtanga Yoga style and philosophy, has taught power yoga. It is also referred to as the western variant of Ashtanga yoga in India.

Power yoga is energetic and aerobic, making it very popular with people.

It works with the mind and experience of the student and brings into action the yoga eight limbs.

Jnana Yoga Jnana means wisdom (sometimes referred to as "Gnana") and is a wise man. Often named the "discernment yogi."

This method of yoga concentrates on the study of the inner life and adhyatmic topics, the practice of some relaxations and contemplative kriyas for contemplation.

The primary aim of jnana meditation is to detach mind and intention from the view of life and self in a deluded fashion so as to see and exist in accordance with truth or spirit.

This style of yoga focuses on meditation to transform and illuminate.

Karma Yoga Karma means "life." "life." Karma Yoga is based on the practice discipline based on Bhagavad Gita's scriptures, a sacred
Hindu scripture.

This yoga of selfless service emphasizes on responsibility (dharma) devotion while staying unrewarded. In this life, as in previous experiences, karma is the cumulative total of our actions.

Bhakti Yoga Bhakti Yoga is performed in several stages. Bhakti means' devotion,' and Guna Bhakti is the intention to worship. A Bhakta Yoga practitioner is not limited to a particular community or religious faith; the path to inner life is more than the strictly devoted.

The selves adore themselves with the same sort.

Bhakti yoga is the situation under which we are in touch with our life and our nature and being. It does not matter whether you believe in it or not. The only attribute is transparency, unforeseen, and uncertain, to the mind and heart.

Many who have read Quantum Mechanics, in which each atom in the world is related to the subordinate truth, would be able to equate this with Bhakti yoga's theory. B.K.S Iyengar, born 14 December 1918 Iyengar Yoga was founded in India. At the age of 16, his Mentor Sri T. Krishnamacharya introduced him to yoga. Iyengar Yoga is also a popular Western model.

Teachers are well aware of the anatomy and the precise position of each pose. Pranayama or the methods of meditation and relaxation are less focused, and hence the practice is common in the west.

Iyengar Yoga focuses more on the correct location of the foot in order to maintain balance with the spine and hips. In their research, Iyengar has developed several various guidance and strategies for individuals.

Other Forms Integral Yoga is a practice of integration, harmonizing the journeys of karma, jnana, and bhakti-yoga. Swami Satchidananda rendered this.

The convergence of Vedanta (Indian philosophical system) and Tantra (Asian concepts and traditions based on the idea of the supreme force forming and sustaining the cosmos, channelling the energy into the human microcosm) is also considered.

It was also clarified as a fusion of spirituality approaches between eastern and western.

Postures are gentler than other yoga types, and lessons typically finish with prolonged intervals of deep relaxation, respiration, and reflection. Integral Yoga is an all-round hatha yoga technique.

Sivananda Yoga Yoga offers a light approach to meditation. Every session involves meditation, praying, and intense relaxation.

Students are urged to be nutritional and vegetarian. Bikrams Yoga is usually taught between 95 and 105 degrees in a bed.

The fire allows muscles and ligaments to relax. There are approximately 26 positions, and this yoga provides proper training due to the extreme sun. This yoga thus emphasizes primarily on the physical execution of postures rather than on the field of relaxing and meditation.

Many of the Big Teachers.

Each style has a growing lineage. The pioneers of two big Raja / Ashtanga / Avenger Yoga models were both students of Krishnamacharya, the same great instructor.

Krishnamacharya Shri T. was born in 1888 in Muchukunte district, state of Karnataka. His formal schooling, primarily in Sanskrit, included graduates from many North Indian universities.

For seven years, he trained in West Tibet with a distinguishable yogi: Rama Mohana Brahmachari, who taught him the therapy of asanas and pranayama. He then returned to South India and set up a yoga school in Mysore's Maharajah palace. He died in 1988 at the age of
101.

Sivananda Yoga and Integral Yoga have both been developed by students of Sivananda, another teacher. Swami Sivananda Saraswati was born in Pattamadai, Tamil Nadu, India. She was born in Kuppuswamy. Born Muslim, he is a well-known follower of yoga and Vedanta (a central branch of Muslim philosophy).

It is recorded that during his lifetime, he has written over 300 books on these and similar subjects. In 1936, he formed the modern "Divine Life Society" religious movement on the banks of the Holy Ganges River. He passed away on 14 July 1963.

AND WHAT TYPE IS RIGHT FOR YOU?

These are not all forms of yoga, but you can tell from each of these brief examples that yoga practice can be radically different.

Growing uses repetitive postures and meditation to stabilize the body, an essential aspect of the yoga method.

This is where it is essential for the student to consider and select a style that fits his or her yoga practice. If you do one and don't think it's enough physical, do another one because it would be totally different if you launch one too difficult to turn around again before you find the lesson.

Some of us just want to work on the body, and others want to concentrate more on a form of self-realization, whatever the cause there are plenty of models to fulfil our needs every day.

You are never too old to continue yoga, people starting for the first time in their seventies and witnessing life's changes. If you have just sat and watched your cat or dog waking up, what are they doing?

Stretch. Stretch. When we pause just for a second to look at what we can know about nature and the animal world, we will notice that even the initial delay was missing somehow when we evolved.

Prepare for the First Yoga

For the first time every year, thousands of people try yoga and forget how to train themselves for their first yoga lesson.

Sometimes, inexperienced students are confused with the fact that they have the right equipment and expertise to prepare for a class before visiting a classroom or a gym to practice yoga.

Below are a few tips for your first session in yoga.

Train your body:

This is a smart guideline any time you exercise. Should not eat 1-3 hours before a workout. Drink water all day long, ensuring that the body is properly hydrated and able to shift and rest.

Materials:

You would want to buy a non-slip yoga mat before your first lesson. Recommendations may be obtained from other graduates, teachers, and sales staff. Wear clothes that are simple, stretchy, and comfortable to walkabout. Try carrying a closed water bottle into the classroom for hydration. Now, when required, hold a rag or sweat towel.

Set up for success: Choosing the right class for your level is one of the easiest ways to practice for your first yoga lesson. Speak to a studio or gym regarding different instructors and courses to find out what one will be best for beginners to take their first yoga lessons.

Using the mind of beginners: many times in our lives, we experience for the first time, something that can be an incredible obstacle both psychologically and physically.

Speak about your first yoga instructor, realizing that this is a new area of research, and possibly, you would make mistakes. Seek to use your instructor's tips and feedback to enhance your first yoga experience on the mat.

Open-minded practice:

Pranayama, meditation, psychology,

Sanskrit, and a number of other techniques, forms, and instruments used in yoga study. Hold your eyes free and know that it may be completely different from something you have ever done.

That is all right! You can discover something different there to improve your mind and body, and occasionally you can feel weird or uncomfortable. It's the first yoga lesson and takes advantage of the chance to learn new stuff.

Trust your instructor:

Listen to your instructor carefully and try to execute the series in the best possible way. Many instructors practice, learn and teach yoga for hundreds of hours. Confidence that even though your first yoga class arrives, they will take care of you.

Especially if you tell an instructor that this is your first lesson, they should pay particular attention to your form and offer assistance or corrections if appropriate.

Follow the appropriate yoga tag:

Particularly, make sure to come early for your first yoga lesson and let the teacher know that you are brand new in yoga. If you are late, enter the room after meditation is opened.

Follow the rest of the sequence as appropriate. The pose of a kid is also an outstanding choice if you need a rest. Relax! In any yoga lesson, but particularly in your first class, it is necessary to concentrate on your breath and link air to movement.

Proper breath or pranayama produces a sense of calmness and emphasizes the awareness and relation in yoga, which lets you understand that everybody returns to yoga after their first lesson.

As this is your first yoga lesson, this will first seem like a challenge, but continue to train and make use of your tissue.

Post-practice routine:

Clean your mat and place the props in the correct cupboards. It will build a rhythm starting from the first class of yoga that will help to minimize the room with every session, if not more.

Tell the instructor some concerns that could have arose during the lecture, as it was a new experience.

Change your clothing and wash if necessary to purify yourself from the exercise.

Take your yoga off the mat:

Talk about the lesson's physical, mental, and emotional effects. It may take a few lessons to realize how the activity impacts you as you may feel confused by new knowledge and experiences during your first yoga session.

Taking your teachings and find ways to bring them into your daily life. Real improvement and progress in each new activity or routine are followed by regular commitment and dedication to specific steps along the way.

No matter what, seek another after your first yoga session! Seek to be optimistic and celebrate the small wins along the way. Yoga is a way of life and has too much to say if you just try it.

YOGA PRESENT AND PAST

Proper yoga practise plays a significant role in achieving optimal physical and mental growth. Each posture has its own benefit.

Others cure back problems, while others have immunity from diseases.

Beginners can have several difficulties doing different yoga movements. We cannot train with absolute consistency and productivity due to a lack of knowledge.

Below are a few tips to improve beginners' practice experience.

- The best equipment–First and foremost, beginners will pick the ideal material to execute their workout. Casual and tight clothing will spoil a workout.

They are not comfortable and smart enough to go to a yoga session. An individual should select a perfect pair of yoga pants and tops before starting his workout. He will review different yoga outfits and choose one that provides optimum comfort.

Mind also that a pant should be loose when the top should be tight. They can also be consumed with unnecessary sweat. Proper wardrobe preference is one of the main stages of successful teaching.

- Essential items to carry - The next thing to remember after finding a great wardrobe is important stuff to carry.

You will bring a pad and a water bottle for a good yoga session. A mat is one of the critical aspects of an exercise. This provides warmth and benefits a lot with both body and mind.

Most courses of yoga have their own mat, so if you train at home, you can pick a carpet with due thought. Even hold a water bottle in your pocket after pad. A cold water bottle can be very convenient for hot and intensive yoga lessons. This will help a lot to will the temperature of the body.

Then remember these things and ensure that you have them before you continue your practice session.

- Proper warmth-The The next aspect to be taken into consideration before beginning a practice session is adequate warmth.

You cannot benefit from different postures without decent warming up. Before you continue, you should warm your body by performing different Suryanamaskar exercises.

The primary positions included in this activity will train you for awkward situations.

- The next thing that should be considered is the creation of an optimistic outlook. A confident and growth-oriented mindset is essential for yoga practice to be successful.

You should keep focused and strive to accomplish the goals to achieve the most significant outcomes. The only way to produce effective and sustainable results is to be committed and to perform best.

Note also the lack of ambition and constructive positivity paves the way for mistakes.

There were some critical tips for beginners in yoga class. After these tips, new practitioners will begin their practice nicely.

Combining both and self-efforts will produce optimal outcomes in the shortest possible period. Regularity is the path to optimal fitness.

The history of Yoga has many positions of secrecy and confusion because of its oral communication of Holy Scriptures and its secret instruction. Yoga's origins can be traced to 5000 years.

The History, The first evidence of Yoga, was uncovered during archeological excavations in the Indus valley where old sculptures show a figure, which some archeologists think, depicts a yogi sitting on a traditional yoga cross-legged posture with his hands on his knees meditating.

Yoga's long and rich history can be categorized into four major evolutionary stages:
- The Vedic
- The Preclassical
- The Classical, and
- The postclassical stages

This era is characterized by the presence of the Vedas. The Vedas contain the earliest known Yoga teachings and are called Vedic Yoga as well. Rituals and rituals that seek to transcend the limits of the spirit reflect this.

The Vedic people relied on the rishis or Vedic yogis at this period to
teach them how to live in spiritual peace.

Pre-Classical Yoga Pre-Classical Yoga is the development of the Upanishads. The Upanishads clarify the Vedas ' teachings.

Yoga has some characteristics that we can follow, not only with Hinduism but also with Buddhism. During the sixth century B.C., Buddha started to teach Buddhism, which underlines the importance of meditation and daily body practice.

Earlier, around 500 B.C. has produced the Bhagavad-Gita or Lord's Song and is the earliest known text of yoga at present.

This is utterly committed to Yoga and has stated that it has been an ancient tradition for a while. Like the Upanishads in the Vedas, the Gita draws on the doctrines present in the Upanishads and integrates them.

The classical era is characterized by another development-the Yoga Sutra. The classical era. Written in the second century by Patanjali, this was an attempt to describe and standardize traditional yoga.

Patanjali believed every person to be a combination of matter and spirit; he found the two must be separated in order to purify the spirit-a direct contrast to Vedic andPre-Classical Yoga, which implies the union of body and mind.

The philosophy of Patanjali existed for several hundred years, so much so that some Yogis focused solely on meditation and ignored the Asanas. Much later was the trust of the body rekindled, and the insistence on the value of the Asana reinvigorated.

A large number of independent yoga schools and styles evolved during the post-yoga sutras era. Like Patanjalis Yoga, the Yoga of this period was characterized by the union of the mind and body, much like the postclassical tradition and the Vedic tradition.

Yogis from the past did not rely much on the (physical) body as they concentrated all their attention on reflection and contemplation.

Nevertheless, the New Generation of Yogis created a method that would serve to keep the body alive and sustained, coupled with deep breathing and meditation. It has opened the way for the development of Hatha Yoga and other Tantra Yoga branches and schools.

To have made a profound impact on America he introduced. Yoga masters continued to move to the west and gained interest and supporters. Throughout the 1920s, throughout India, Hatha Yoga was actively advocated with T's lifetime work. Krishnamacharya.

Krishnamacharya travelled through India to demonstrate yoga poses and opened the Hatha Yoga School for the first time.

In the 1950s, one of H.E. Selvarajan Yesudian, one of the leading practitioners of yoga in his day, wrote a book entitled "Sport and Yoga."

Today we will see numerous sports teams and athletes who use yoga in their lesion prevention, rehabilitation and centred fitness schemes.

Yoga now, Yoga has grown immensely, has more than 30 million participants from all over the world, and is today's fastest-growing fitness phenomenon.

All now know the physical and mental benefits of yoga from celebrity to common man; in addition, many doctors prescribe yoga, particularly for stress and relaxation.

People have shifted their views towards wellbeing, morality, way
of life, and our place in society very dramatically. When we suffer from physical and psychological pain steadily, and battle new and old ailments, yoga does also seem to be a friend's solution.

THE SAFE YOGA

Safe yoga has the following characteristics:
- Secure (instructor, environment, and student).
- Consciousness (to measure, quantity, poses, form).
- Functional (diligent study options, offers improvements).
- Active (provides versatility, user-friendliness, strength, and balance).

Yoga is more common than ever before. Why come? Why come? Yoga offers full exercise that boosts strength, endurance, flexibility, and versatility.

Therefore, it increases one's consciousness, strengthens muscle strength, and promotes dominance of the body.

Since this requires an extremely detailed and streamlined process, yoga produces a faster, sleeker, and more fluid physics.

Yoga also allows you to relieve stress and fatigue through mindfulness, often-fluid motion, and a strong focus on breathing.

When teachers do not follow the UNIQUE criteria of the environment of the Health Club and its clients, unintended accidents can occur.

Traditional yoga no longer exists in the US, but yoga exercise models are ideal for gyms-it is quite necessary.

Healthy Yoga is unlike traditional yoga since the poses are fluidly heat generating. Breath is connected with movements that naturally and chemically burn your body.

Whenever possible, rest is encouraged.

Warm-ups are particularly necessary because exercise rooms usually are new. Warm the body up thoroughly with full-body motions before engaging in some dynamic or fluid pose.

Health and wellness activities such as sit-ups, push-ups, drop, and keep are combined. Transitions are seamless, from posture to stance with a complete focus on body training; all areas of the bodywork similarly.

Adjustments and sizes can be made to accommodate the needs of numerous students in different regions of the room. Teachers teach of OR, Par, MODIFY, forcing students to split, LET GO perceptions, judgment, and rivalry, and never push their own limits beyond. Teachers will never make violent physical changes to their students.

Community fitness teachers will begin by incorporating yoga poses into their own current lessons; step, spin, kickbox, and aerobics.

It provides the ability to help you with a few simple Roles-Respond to these critical questions before recruiting an instructor:
- Do you know the AFAA and ACE Contraindications Health Guidelines?
- Will you know how yoga is related?
- You underwent a formal Yoga Instructor Practice.
- Were you happy with the positions?
- Are you confident with the poses?
- Have you a regular practice of yoga?

If you replied yes to all of the above, then it is time to continue. Hear these men!

A professional attitude in the health club is not a suitable type.

Look for a personal trainer who is first and foremost, teaching a private teacher in yoga is much better than educating a conventional yoga instructor in exercise.

Courses Formatting: If the instructor chooses poses in your current training or a good yoga lesson, a period of the warm-up is expected.

Much like we don't flex before exercise, we don't want to take complicated yoga poses until our body is moist and comfortable to go.

A minimum of 5 minutes of yoga breathing will begin each lesson. It helps clear your mind and makes your body happy. The air intake is also the most critical aspect of our yoga exercise.

Inhaling and inhaling the nose hold the moisture in your body and concentrates your thoughts. The most reliable foundation on which we develop our yoga practice is deep rhythmic breathing. Teachers have to go back regularly to maintain genuinely and also ask students to do the same.

Rest and rehabilitation are an essential part of the real yoga, so we relax at the end of the lesson at least five minutes to rejuvenate, refresh so bring back the body.

Giving space: The majority of health and exercise coaches do not
have the luxury of separate lighting and heating power.

Healthy Yoga is an ideal option for the wellness and fitness community. If the lights are dark at all times, turn off the Air-con and pick up energy yoga videos.

In addition to other specialized programs, including Boys, PreNatal, Senior and this style of yoga provides four types of teacher instruction. This provides an extensive line of online instructional guides for teachers, clubs, and pupils.

We also teach hatha yoga exercises with a focus on training study. For all the success of yoga, numerous accidents have arisen, and this form of yoga sees the need for anatomy and preparation to prepare better yoga teachers and exercise practitioners so that yoga pupils obtain amazing yoga stuff without the risks.

YOGA OF PRE-NATAL

Pre-natal yoga involves activities and breathing techniques that make labour a lovely and less stressful experience. Preparing for motherhood is the best thing any woman might do. The old art of yoga, which originates in the Orient, is no longer an exclusive right east of the globe.

There are currently more exponents of yoga in the west than in the east. Mothers will also have access to some of the several online and offline pre-natal yoga workout programs.

When you are not especially interested in going outside, you can pick either of the program's online models.

The scheme deals with more than just a selection of yoga workouts specifically chosen for mother-to-be; the course, practically, encompasses anything from nutritional recommendations to medication guidelines.

The holistic approach is not just suited during the third quarter of pregnancy. It makes you physically and emotionally well prepared for the new process that is about to take place.

Pre-natal yoga sessions are performed by professionals and individuals actively interested in the scientific community. You should be assured that the instructions and workouts recommended are in accordance with the body and baby needs.

A number of women in the world swear by the program's performance. There is a range of tools that encourage your partner to take part in the joy of exercising while at the same time taking on additional responsibilities mentally.

The movements are discreet, gentle, and ideal for turning the body into action.

Breathing techniques should be performed even in the office.

Physicians who perform symposia for pregnant women have prenatal yoga instruction as a required part of their preparation.

The exercises now provide a host of options to needing you to take into account the portion, time schedule, and dietary components to keep you light and safe and yet nutritious.

Both services are tailored to protect your health and well-being and provide you with a well-rounded and conscientious lifestyle.

The practice of yoga becomes very quick to understand and is an integral part of your life. Prenatal yoga is the perfect way for you to prepare for your surprises and during the post-natal years.

The slow rhythmic motions relax the mind with every step. This meditation concentration allows you to have a strong bond between mind and body.

It is a vital aspect of the work and distribution process. This helps you to relax and be calm in a challenging environment otherwise.

The breathing exercises used during your yoga practice will only give you the bond between your mind and body you would require, but also give you the strength to resolve your hard labor.

The kegel exercises, which come so highly recommended show you what muscles you use when the time is right to move.

The two different things can be achieved so quickly that each of your work through concurrently. Yes, poses and movements move with the wind in yoga. This helps to create a link between mind and body and encourages you to concentrate on a particular area of the body.

In this scenario, you would like to concentrate on the so-called pelvic floor. They are the muscles that keep you from going to the bathroom, all right, what you are doing. All right.

"Ew" does not seem to be doing it for others, but honestly, it helps.

Minor exercise to try out with you. When the muscles that prevent you from going to the toilet have been found, you are ready for the next step, Kegels.

Lie in a quiet position with as little pressure as possible on the pelvic region (if that is even practicable at this point in your pregnancy).

Take a couple of deep breaths. At the next inhale, the pelvic floor muscles will be lined up by varying degrees. Imagine putting those muscles up a stair run. Upon the exhalation, muscles are released in quick steps, or muscles are carried down the stairs.

The gradual deep breaths, along with the concentration brace the mind for the amount of effort and execution needed. So the intention of the exercises in kegel? In order to recognize the muscles, you drive.

Once you expel the flesh, such are the muscles and the feeling with which you need to know yourself and brace for the big move.

Millions of women who have studied yoga during pregnancy have shown that it can help ready the body for conception. Support your body plan for the big event with yoga as a prenatal workout.

CHAPTER TWO

The Yoga Process

Since you can do yoga at any time, many people like to do just after they wake up and before they go to bed. Unless you want to train more in a classroom environment, you have to wait until the class is in session.

The first thing in the morning is to do a yoga practice is a perfect way to wake you up and set your goals for the day.

Also, if you will only leave 20 minutes before you head to work to have the children up for the day, you would be well prepared for the day.

Ideally, the evening before you go to bed, you ought to have a yoga session. This can help you remove all the pressures and acts accrued from the day so that you can get a happier and healthier night.

There could also be perfect opportunities all day long, where you can add to your mini yoga exercises to help relieve any painful or traumatic activities-5 to 10 minutes would allow you to handle it even in the shower!

When possible, it is best to alleviate tension more quickly, so that it does not linger in your body and will accumulate up over time and potentially develop infections that you do not like.

Yoga will contribute to the escape of life by concentrating your attention on Yoga here and now, but you would always continue to strengthen yourself and achieve optimum benefits for body, mind, and spirit.

The easiest way to maintain and sustain your relaxation is to have it in your daily routine. The trick is listening to your body when practicing yoga so you can get the most out of it and know what is right for your organization.

The process of calming the body's muscles gives relaxation to the collection and the mind. Through practice, you are reliable, agile, and balanced, and Yoga helps you build symmetry around the body.

Yoga is a perfect way to build a balanced body and mind.

Yoga increases your endurance, general health, and makes your mind and body calmer. Yoga has also been a source of many wellbeing benefits for both the mind and the body.

Thanks to the close link between mind and body in yoga, daily yoga practice has multiple emotional benefits.

There are many different yoga forms around the world. Bikram yoga and Hatha yoga are two of the most common styles of yoga.

Hatha Yoga is the most traditional type of yoga in the World;

Bikram Yoga is better done for those who want to do heat yoga, which is good for muscle and joint injuries, as long as you do not have high blood pressure or heat sensitivity. In recent decades, yoga has become very popular here in the West.

Yoga postures and relaxation exercises and breathing techniques can help you learn to relieve muscle tension and calm the body.

Kids will learn to rest, pacing, calming, and focusing. Older people are relatively healthy because' life gets in the way' or start learning how to change the physical disabilities that arise, as you get older.

Athletes may practise yoga to improve their capacity to either prevent injuries or either heal from injuries that have occurred.

The journey begins as the body revitalizes by movement, breathing, and relaxation. With its emphasis on absolute, purifying breathing, deep breath is an easy and effective technique for relaxation. The main modes of respiration are normal, abdominal, and reverse abdominal.

The gentle stretching reduces muscle and joint tension and rigidity as well as rising strength.

Prenatal Yoga is generally very healthy during pregnancy and a perfect way to get in touch and brace for conception.

Ashtanga Yoga practises should be adjusted during pregnancy to accommodate the growing baby and preserve the placenta. Most women cannot wait until they return to fertility, particularly after their first baby is born.

Prenatal Yoga is a great way to train for conception and can help moms in shape before and during pregnancy. During birth, workouts should be modified to suit women at all times. Final relaxation is an essential factor in maternity practice and an excellent time to communicate with your infant.

Yoga health, there are many different yoga forms, and although many are safe, they may be challenging, and they may not be ideal for everyone.

The trick is to be careful of what your body tells you when you practice yoga and to be sure you breathe.

Short, quick respirations won't give you the strength you need and won't help you alleviate pain and tightness. When working on a task, make sure you breathe through tight or stressed muscles.

Then let it out. Just let it out. You tend to improve tightness by breathing in so that as you breathe out, you feel the tension absorbed in the muscles, joints, and areas of the body. This takes time to learn this.

However, it is also worth it because then almost every day, you will relieve tightness.

The least 10 to 20 minutes. A Day A yoga practice may take from 20 to 90 minutes and may be performed with a teacher at home or at work.

There is a start, a middle, and a finish of every class and every session. While students can start a session anytime, a session course allows more consistency, particularly for beginners.

You should exercise self-compassion anywhere in your day, even though you only have 15 or 30 seconds.

The muscles and tissues that accompany each injury the yoga cycle includes relaxing and strengthening muscles. You have to use precisely, methodically, and mathematically to measure how you will lie, how you can write, how you can stretch your neck.

A problematic solution is not to try to worry that will drag you out, but to help you land, rejuvenate to free up. Your role is to be there, and not to do anything consciously.

The muscles are forced to stretch and gradually lengthen without rapid movements, which triggers tears and muscles.

Recall the yoga is smooth and versatile. Some are likely to feel closer or more stressed than most.

You want to be able to change your routine if necessary so that you can experience less harm. Although yoga is a reasonably safe exercise and is often used to help you heal from injuries caused by other activities, you can injure yourself. Just be careful what the body tells you.

If the trainer suggests that the body cannot do it, do not do it. Shift the task of what you can do or ask the instructor what else you can do. It's all right to be unique.

HOW CAN IT HELP YOU?

Yoga has many benefits for its consumers. There are medically many conditions, which can benefit from yoga detox. Yoga is, however, often meant to merge mind, body, and spirit and bring numerous other healing advantages of yoga.

Consider only a few ways in which yoga has proven incredibly beneficial. The various positions used in yoga call for multiple joints that are rarely worked or even heard.

Using these joints during yoga will help to improve strength for individuals.

Yoga positions are excellent preparation for tendons and ligaments when exercising the joints. Even areas of the body where you do not work consciously benefit from adjustable yoga positions.

This will improve the lubrication of the muscles, ligaments, and tendons by yoga practice. There are many parts of the body that receive no external stimuli during their lifespan. Yoga is perhaps the best way to relax all the inner glands and organs of the body through the different poses.

The various parts of the body receive some form of regular yoga exercise, which helps keep diseases away and lets individuals recognize when their body is likely to be affected.

Extension during yoga practice allows the body's muscles, joints, and various organs to be massaged and to ensure the maximum blood flow for all areas of the body.

The enhanced blood flow serves to extract the toxins from a person's bloodstream and fuel other areas of the body. A slower aging cycle, improved vitality, and a healthy mental outlook on life can provide the benefits of this blood flow.

Yoga is not an intense workout, but it gives an ideal way to relax muscles. Some flaccid or weak muscles can be quickly toned with yoga that helps to lose excess pounds and improve the skin look contributing to youth. It shows that yoga has advantages both outdoors and inside.

When comparing the advantages of yoga with physical exercise, you can clearly understand how yoga is the perfect way to find a way to sustain a balanced mind and body. Yoga relies on the parasympathetic nervous system, while the sympathetic nervous system is usually used for certain types of meditation.

The distinction allows yoga to concentrate on the brain's subcortical regions, while other types focus only on the brain's frontal zones.

Yoga concentrates on the implementation of steady, static, and fluid motions to achieve benefits when most other methods of exercise involve quick and energetic movements that can lead to health issues when performed wrongly.

Yoga contributes to muscle tone normalization, while fitness raises muscle stress.

Yoga positions include a style of exercise that has a low chance of damaging the muscles and ligaments. In contrast, certain other forms of exercise, mainly if incorrectly carried out, can be at higher risk of injury.

You concentrate on low-calorie intake in yoga, but you do require moderate to high caloric consumption with certain types of exercise to maintain the stamina for your workout. The yoga cycle involves little preparation and allows a balanced fitness system for the body.

Many other workouts require full commitment and high stress. The standard and regulated respiration in yoga increase the sense of relaxation when the forced inhalation of certain types of exercise also leaves you exhausted.

Yoga is a process-oriented, non-competitive way to work out your body. It concentrates on a coordinated movement with competing muscle groups and focuses on internal consciousness by breathing.

Yoga does not hinder the development of your self-awareness.
Most frequently than not, other types of competition are aggressive and goal-oriented, with an imbalanced activity focused on competing muscle groups. External knowledge is at the heart of the goal-oriented approach, and the consideration is that you will quickly be disturbed by the techniques engaged in this kind of exercise.

Simple Ways To Jump Begin Your Health

Over recent years, yoga has been a staple in the west as a way to boost people's health. However, many people are still skeptical that yoga will offer them benefits. The best yoga poses for beginners and each one's advantages.

Oh, what's the essence of poses in yoga? The various poses were created to help people maintain improved health and well-being by alleviating pain and discomfort around the body.

Throughout the years, ' many yoga masters have mastered and adjusted the poses so that nearly everyone can put their poses into their routine and reap enormous health benefits with just a few minutes a day.

- Balancing in Yoga, their equilibrium starts to deteriorate as people mature. The risk of injury due to poor coordination and stance may be enhanced.

A right balance is required, particularly in older people, to maintain a good posture. The use of balancing positions in yoga can at first be a little confusing, but once you get the hang of these positions, the attitude can improve.

- In Yoga, you can try some sitting positions in yoga to improve the strength of your hips and lower back. You should also improve the back muscles by using these poses.

You should even breathe slowly, allowing the body the extra oxygen it requires to function correctly.

- Standing positions in yoga, Exercises in balance with the body are very useful in yoga.

By doing these standing positions, you strengthen your stance and flexibility by gently relaxing your back and chest.

Through proper balance, you can even remove any back issues that might be normal over the years. Standing poses help you sculpt your muscles and make your thighs and hips more flexible.

This was a basic description of the three basic yoga poses for newbies. Only note that every posture has its benefits for enhancing your body and health. You will first find that it is difficult to perform any of these poses, but if you stick to them, you will be able to learn them in no time.

YOGA POSES FOR RUNNERS, CYCLISTS, AND TRIATHLETES

This illustrates that yoga asanas support riders, triathletes, and runners with tight muscles effectively.

If you are running or cycling a lot, you also have steep legs. This rigidity of the legs, from the foot to the gluteus point, will lead to various complications, including, for example, the iliotibial band syndrome. Many issues caused by weak leg muscles are back injuries. Back problems. For more posts on knee issues and their avoidance, please search my blog.

These poses are particularly perfect for yoga beginners. It allows you to keep your legs more comfortable. Growing asana is defined in English and Sanskrit to encourage you to find videos and images of the poses on the web or on a book.

You can work with less effort because the muscles are more stable.
You can drive or spin more quickly. This can also help to avoid overuse of iliotibial band syndrome injuries.

Once you continue to do yoga or rest, you will no longer have knee pain.

To beginners, it is common to experience a slight feeling of pain as they attempt to get into the different asanas. Don't give up! Don't give up!

With daily stretching, you can achieve stability to get into postures much better. You will just enjoy them at the end.

Triangle Pose: It is an adorable pose for the thighs. Holding forward (Uttanasana): This posture flexes all your hamstrings, your maximal gluteus, your screen, your minimus, and your spinal muscles.

People with back injuries will be cautious about this curve. Gravity, don't put your body in the picture, will do the job. When the hamstrings are very high, it is advised to bend your knees. This is going to increase the gap.

Warrior I: Warrior I is a reliable place to apply hip flexors to other riders and cyclists who are poor. It improves hip, back, and frontal strength.

Warrior II (Virabhadrasana II): It is another hip joint pose. This also strengthens the groins and extends the inner muscles of the leg.

Pose Side Angle: Stretches the back of the legs and extends the neck. This also covers the upper body. Is an excellent Warrior II associate.

Triangle Pose (Trikonasana): Warrior I stance follow-up. There, above all, the buttocks work together.

Intense side stretch (Parsvottanasana): This operates on the best of the hamstrings and gluteus. This offers you a better time for your hamstrings than in the forward curve that stands.

Broad forward bent (Prasarita Padottanasana): It is an excellent asana to stretch the hamstrings and full gluteus. The distinction is that in this place, you have your feet further apart. This is often referred to as a big leg forward fold.

To make the most of the asanas mentioned above, remain in place for five deep breaths. You raise your vagina regularly and increase the strength of your legs and hips. This reduces the risk of issues caused by overuse.

If you do the asanas at least three days a week and do it for two months, we will be able to hit the next point.

Yoga Beginners Poses

If you do not find yoga now, it can be very daunting to see any of the more advanced yoga poses. Nonetheless, note that everybody should do yoga before you dismiss yoga as something you cannot do.

Including young children to elderly adults, yoga is perfect for all. This is an old tradition that includes physical postures, calming breathing exercises, and deep meditation to unite the mind, body, and spirit as one.

Often yoga practitioners develop a profound sense of knowledge of themselves and the world. Yoga may sound very distant to the untrained person, but if you practice these poses, you can find that yoga is an enjoyable and healed activity that can be incorporated into the health care program.

Below are some starting positions to get you on your yoga ride. The Dog Pose is good with a safe neck.
Dog and Cat Pose This is ideal for beginners as it has small impacts and is not as taxing physically as other yoga poses. Begin by standing on your knees and hands. Place your hands above your shoulders slightly.

Respire gradually and upward the tailbone and pelvis. To do so correctly, you should raise your chin, lower your butt, and bend your spine
downwards. Stretch this pose as long as you can without question.

Going into the cat pose by exhaling and rotating the spot, bending the spine upward and downward. Do these places as much as you can?

Future Bends this exercise aims to enhance and develop the stability of arms and legs. Stand right in front of your face with your palms touching (Mountain Pose).

Uplift your palms high over your head while you inhale. Bend on your knees on the exhale and drop your back to the ground. If possible, bend your knees and make sure your hands hit the surface. Slowly climb up the next inhalation and repeat the exhalation. Allow four to five loops to experience the impact.

Cobra Pose It is a perfect pose for stretching your back and body. Start your posture by lying flat with your arms near your chest and feet securely together. Start lifting your head and shoulders as high as possible, while keeping the breathing rhythm steady and slow.

Brace your body with your hands and bend your buttocks. Hold this pose for roughly 30 seconds and return to exhalation. Go back up and keep the spot again.

The Cobra Pose helps to reinforce the back muscles and make them more mobile. Corpse Pose Normally, the stance to complete all the yoga exercises is a perfect way to unwind after a workout, and it feels fantastic.

Start by lying flat on your back with your feet slightly apart, palms upwards with your arms on your hands. Breathe a couple of deep breaths.

Be mindful of the pressures in your body, and seek to calm as you fall into the mat. Free your mind from distractions and focus on relaxing. Hold this pose for about ten minutes to feel calm and relaxed during your yoga session.

For thousands of years, Yoga has been with us, and how it still can be seen as a phenomenon so far is always amazing!

Since it has been done for such a long time, it has grown at such a slow pace.

For this cause, the growing types of yoga today, mostly with comfortable cushioned pushes, stretching pants, and lots of gestures, are virtually modern.

Such innovations tend not to vitiate Yoga's conventional physical focuses (asanas). In fact, practising yoga is now delivering better outcomes from a yoga activity that is more than practical for the least evolving, solid, stable bodies. Yoga activities will require, at some level, a relaxed, open mind and spiritual illumination.

Nonetheless, it is appropriate to initiate a yoga practice for some occasion. And this exercise, like everything else, should always begin with the basics. And so, for beginners, yoga poses will start with these five simple poses.

Broad Leg Forward Fold or Prasarita Padottanasana. This style will first create a little discomfort for beginners who have tight hamstrings.

This role may be rendered in multiple models, but does not mean that hands or head-to-floor modes will be used automatically. Experiencing the body's apparent activities is more important as the exercise continues than getting to a particular position or form fast.

Move into the right form: stand wide open on your mat with the hands-on your hips. Shoulder blades will be on the collar and come together. The feet will still be kept parallel.

Try to imagine your foot as a brace, with your eyes closed, with one point on your heel, the other under your big toe on the pad, and the other under your little toe. Root all three points into the earth.

Inhale slowly and imagine that you take the roots from the position under your toes to your hips. This will potentially trigger your leg muscles and allow you to maintain the right balance.

Exhale, fold your body on your shoulders while holding your back straight. Bring your hands on the ground if you can afford it. Do so as the back is stretched.

When you cannot quite touch the ground, bend your legs and your palms on your thighs. As you hold this position, a few priorities must be met.

Your spine must also be kept long, or stretched-this facilitates a more substantial back balance and strength and will help avoid lower back injuries.

It is essential to preserve the tripods planted on the ground. From these points comes the energy shown in this physical shape–this encourages the energy of the feet, proper leg balance that avoids injuries, and keeps you safe when in poses.

Downward Dog, The most popular method of yoga, is applauded. Yet it could be far more complicated than anyone could imagine. It is also a form that stretches the hamstrings.

It may also be a strengthener of the leg, back, and neck.

You can use your entire body, and you can consciously get into it.

Stand on the mat with the feet parallel and hip-width.

Much as the first one, plant again the tripod.

Inhale your hand and raise it to the stars.

Exhale. Exhale. Fold your hips over so you can place your hands on the concrete, and brace your knees if necessary.

Take a step back so you can create an upside-down a V. (This is the fundamental pose.) Note: it is essential that you have a long and straight spin from the knees.

So it's your goal to stretch your back, and it's all right to bend your knees.
St your legs as much as you can into the width of the back.

Keep the feet to the wall; do not lift them as high as possible. They're trying to get there.

You should place your fingertips and pads squarely on the table. It will potentially wear your arm off while shielding it.

Recall that all will be coordinated. Feet should be held straight, and hands should match the shoulder.

Crescent Pose Crescent Pose in most yoga classes is the most favoured beginning form. Either they are trained with flows or other complicated forms or poses.

The fundamental shape of the crescent pose is a forward-standing lung with arms spread overhead.

Choose the perfect shape: From the forward turn, rotate your right leg, fold onto your left leg for some time.

Take your time with your lung recovery. Ensure sure that your feet are straight, your legs solid and your back stretched. You should drop your back knee to the ground if you choose.

Inhale your hand and raise your body to your front knees. If the formation feels right, try to lift your arms over your head with the palm faced in the next inhale.

Push your heart out and then bring your shoulder blades down on your back to add a back end. Whenever the standing lung is still challenging, take the first step back to the lung and drop the back of the knee to the ground.

Warrior II Warrior poses can be used in yoga as a favourite. And Warrior II may be one of the most common variants.

Officially, there are three standing fighters, other improvements have been made, and there are many more pairs of sitting positions. When to get into the right pose: Take a step back from your forward fold into a long lung.

Twist your back foot when you move horizontally so that it's flat on the floor parallel to your mat. Be sure that the feet are set squarely on the table.

Inhale the legs for a strong foundation when drawing power. Extend your limbs to your sides as you raise your upper body straight to match the surface.

Look past the middle finger and breathe slowly before you.

Remember: The secret to a mighty warrior is a stable base. Hold your feet embedded in the earth while you apply power to your legs. It will allow you to accurately balance your position and give you consistency.

The rear will be pushed off and off. Your shoulder could roll forward, let it move forward. Stretch your body to your knees. Warriors don't have flopping wings.

The look you must have is a critical and not a natural aspect of the picture. This can be difficult for us to keep our eyes focused without distracting it and not allowing it to roam about. You need to concentrate on a fighter as he needs to breathe at his presence in the same place.

Child's Pose or Balasana, another form of yoga for beginners, is the pose of an infant. It can be a stage where you can take a rest or cool down. In a yoga session, whenever you want to take a rest, you are allowed to take this role. This acts as a break in a lesson, whether required or part of the curriculum.

Get into it: Kneel, then lean over. Turn. Arrive before you before your knees hit the table.

You can put a block or a roll-up blanket over your calves, or where
you like, or a blanket under your knees, if it's hard to kneel.

When it's difficult to plant your forward to the ground, your hands can serve as block support.

Relax all your muscles, then concentrate on your breath. This shape is not an office, but a relaxing massage. And, if you're ever exasperated, you will change the role.

Yoga may be complicated at first, but everything works as you would wish, with little patience on the line!

CHAPTER THREE

Yoga Poses For The Flexibility

Did you ever wonder how versatile other people are, and you're, yeah, not?

If you're new to yoga, it can be really daunting when you see someone doing a whole split while sitting there thinking how you can even begin to overcome the role.

Okay, for a moment, let me be honest with you. Some people are already resilient, and others (including me) only have to try a little harder to obtain such outcomes.

Don't think agile people are quick, they still have hurdles to solve, just as you do when you conquer this one!

But some of the people you believe are easily bendy don't necessarily just put a lot of hard work and attention to their targets.

Consistency and concentration are the secrets to achieving the
outcomes you seek.

Despite trying one time and failing, you can't only give up. Offer more credit to yourself than that!

You, too, can accomplish your goals, and when you start, it's daunting. No idea which yoga poses would enhance versatility until switched to more advanced poses.

Yoga poses to boost versatility. Hips, Shoulders, Back, and Hamstrings. Sought to render as many combinations for beginners as possible to help you develop your versatility comfortably and effectively!

SHOULDERS

It is very reasonable for people to have discomfort and tenderness on their shoulders because of weak balance and excessive sitting. For freeing up the shoulders, arms, and surrounding areas like the back, the following poses are perfect.

Pose Eagle Weapon (Garurasana).

Eagle wings supply all shoulders with an extended length. The posture seen here is Eagle's seated version.

You don't have to stack your legs if you have narrow knees, you can easily sit or stand comfortably while practicing eagle.

- Begin by sitting or standing and place the arms in the location that you go and shape 90-degree angles on either side. Be sure that your elbows fit your shoulders.

- Continue pulling your arms in and putting your right arm behind your left arm, so that the right elbow is placed on the left elbow inside.

- Wrap your left arm around your right arm as much as you can, striving to reach the inside of your right elbow when you can't make it all the way, that's all right.

- Press your arms around each other and lift them up to the shoulder level vigorously.

Change: If you can't do the Eagle wings, that's all right. Instead of reaching for contact with your palms, just let your hand take your wrist or forearm, as long as you feel the stretch!

Button (Dhanura). Button.

Bow pose covers the whole front body and is particularly perfect for those who sit at a desk all day long and prefer to hunch because all is drawn downwards, while the back is reinforced.

This can sound overwhelming, but there is a secure method you can use to do it correctly and efficiently and show you the excellent advantages.

How to make Bow Pose:

- Start your belly with your hands facing up and palms to your arms. Bend your knees and bring your feet as low to your ass as possible.

- Get back and grab your ankles with your fingertips.

- Whether you don't have a yoga harness or if you don't have one, you should use a blanket or a lightweight towel.

- Pick your legs slowly off the floor and take your shoes off your feet. It raises your arms automatically and draws your head down.

Modification: When you are using a harness, loop the yoga harness around your ankles and use your palms to grasp the strap, instead of reaching out with your palms.

- Make sure the gap between the knees and thighs is not more significant than hip-width for the length of this pose.

- Make sure that your hands and head are balanced away from your face.

- Double, on the other hand, by rotating the lower neck.

(Setu Bandha Sarvangasana) Bridge.

Although Bridge Pose is well known for its positive effect on the treatment of back pain, it is also an excellent pose for your shoulders!

To bring your hands higher in this position, you should brace your palms and shoulder blades for the length of your pose and not leave your arms and hands flat on the surface. Only holding your hands on the board.

It is a bit more sophisticated version, but if you aren't ready yet, it would still be an excellent idea if you actually put your hands on the table!

How to View Bridge:

- To make a bridge, lie flat on the floor with your legs bent. Be sure they are isolated from the inner hip distance.

- Raise your shoulder blades up enough behind you. Bring your feet to your knees on your shoes as soon as you can.

- Hold your arms and hands flat on the ground on your sides. Raise the next breath slowly from your pelvis, leaving your feet and hands planted. Make a deliberate attempt to keep your hands on the surface.

- Lift your legs during the entire pose, either firmly clamping your hands or pressing them to the table.

Change: When your shoulders are too heavy to pull together your legs, feel free to place them in the mat or pick up a yoga strap and use it for slowly linking your brains while gripping the strap.

Cobra (Bhujangasana).

Cobra Pose is a relaxed stance suitable for beginners who want to strengthen the strength of their shoulders and raise their arms.

It's essential to ensure that you don't overdo the backbend, as it can strain your back.

What to do Pose Cobra:

- Start down to the ground with your knees face down and your hands reaching beneath your arms. Kiss your body in your hands. Kiss your neck.

- Behind you, your thighs should be stretched apart, within the hip-width divided, and your feet should be flat on the ground.

- Take a deep breath and then move your hands into your chest on your next breath.

- Move the feet, pelvis, hands and so that they are balanced and uniformly spread.

Modification: Stretch your legs wider if you feel discomfort in your back when you take this position. You don't have to get into maximum cobra, sit there if you notice a break in Baby Cobra.

Water (Matsyasan).

Fish poses are used as alternative poses for reversals like shoulder hold and plow poses regardless of how great the arms are to be extended.

How to handle fish:

- Start with flat legs on your back on the floor and your hands on your arms.

- Lift your pelvis gently and slip your hands beneath your ass.

- Upon the initial exhalation, lower the forearms into the floor and raise your scapulas out of the floor as you lift your head and abdomen.

- You can keep your backbone as soft as you can, but make sure your forearms are positioned to stretch your elbow.

Change: Feel free to put a block below your back for extra help. For this scenario, instead of holding them at your feet, you should stretch your arms widely.

HIPS

Tight hips are one of the most common concerns of people who start with yoga first. You do not know that you have narrow hips until you see that you can't do those positions, like a yogic squat or a pigeon position.

Mouse (Kapotasana).

Pigeon Pose is perfect for stretching your hip flexors, and it's also a fantastic way to ease the anxiety.

Make sure you take deep inhalation and exhalation in this place to get full benefits and relieve all the energy.

Pigeon Pose What to Do:

- Begin with Downward Facing Dog and then raise the right leg up into the air.

- Click in your middle your right leg and slip it into the back of your right hand.

- The more you move your foot (making your leg parallel to your mat), the further you hit the knee, so conform to your body's comfort. Make sure your right foot is bent to cover your ankle.

- The left knee on the floor will be untucked and bent inwardly.

- Place the hands-on both sides of the legs and take a second to ensure that your weight is equally spread across both thighs.

- You may opt to stand here by your shoulders, on the floor next to your knees, or to a more profound point, gradually fold the adjustment

Forward: if the complete pigeon position is not feasible, it might be appropriate for you to make the corner of your leg less painful. Continue to place a block underneath the hip to could the pressure, but also have a decent stretch.

Cow Face Forward (Adho Mukha Gomukhasana).

It is a perfect stance that gives you a deep stretch in your thighs and a fantastic position for people who have Sciatica.

You can either tie your arms or simply place your hands on the floor when you fold. The secret is the hands.

Cow Face Forward Bend:

- Start in the place of the seated Staff Pose.

- Cross your right leg to the left and bend both legs and drop down to your thighs.

- You should place your right knee at the top of your left now.

- Stand upright and put your hands on your feet. You may either tie your hands behind your back or slip them between your legs and spread them over your legs slowly.

- In one of your hips, you can experience a massive stretch. Make sure you replicate this posture. On the other hand, to keep your body balance.

Change: Do not feel the need to tie your wrists, and you can only pull them off before you. Sometimes, aim to stack your thighs if you cannot stack your knees due to tight hips.

Broad legged forward sitting folds (Upavistha Konasana).

Folding yoga poses have so many advantages in themselves, but Long Legged Seated Forward Fold is particularly fantastic to hit the hips thanks to its extended position.

How to use significant legged forward seated folding:

- Start in Pose Workers. Stretch the legs as long as you can while keeping your seat relaxed.

- Flex all ankles and make sure you raise your legs straight up on the ceiling.

- Push your arm upward with a straight back until you slowly fold into the middle and extend your hands in the opposite direction.

- It's all right, and if you can't reach your toes here, you can always contact your toes or shines.

Change: Use a cushion or pad before you to offer further comfort if it's tough to ply your torso.

Lung Crescent (Anjaneyasana).

You notice the stretch instinctively, and the easiest way is to control the strength of the time with how far you lean over.

Crescent Lunge How to Do:

- Start your knees and then move your left leg to the ground flat with your foot. Untuck your left feet. Untuck your legs.

- Guide your overhead arms as you move your shoulders forward and sink into your left knee.

- When you do, bend your back slightly and raise your arms.

- If that's too hard for you, consider putting your left foot on both hands and use them to step forward slowly.

- Make sure this section, on the other hand, is replicated. Note, take it gently and relax in trouble to relieve all the pain!

Change: Put your palms on your knees for support and to monitor the strength of the stretch better. This also helps to breathe in this position if you find it really awkward.

Three-Legged Dogs (Eka Pada Adho Svanasana)

It is similar to Downward Face Dog, in that you raise a leg into the air, which is the word "Three-Legged." Often it's just called "one-legged horse," since you can have one limb.

How to do three-legged dogs:

- Start in the Facing Dog Downward.

- And sure that your weight is evenly spread across your whole body. If you feel an immense pressure on your shoulders, you'll know that you're not.

- If that is the case, try to touch your heart and move your heels up.

- When you're grounded, raise your right leg straight into the air as far as possible on the next exhalation.

- You'll see your right hip expand right away. For a longer stretch, try to extend your right leg and raise your pelvis to the right of the space and shift your foot to the left of the chest.

Modification: When you put more weight into your upper body, aim to raise the upper body using two yoga blocks between your legs, and concentrate more on the opening section of this pose.

HAMSTRINGS

Whether you're an athlete, at a desk, or new to yoga, you're most definitely hamstrings. Implement poses so importantly to relieve tight hamstrings as tight hamstrings can cause another discomfort, such as lower back pain.

Simple legged forward sitting fold (Paschimottanasana).

Another folding forward sitting posture, but when you do this one, you'll look totally different. Mainly in your hamstrings, you can feel the pull.

How to do straight-legged forward sitting folding:

- Start in place of the staff and rotate both feet.

- Shift some added skin to the hand such that you lie squarely on the sits.
- Lift up your shoulders, spread your legs slowly to touch your knees, ankles or shins.

Change: a harness will be very helpful to get into the gap further and get the most gain. Place it around your foot and take the strap and move your hands on the rope to make the stretch longer.

The Wall of the Legs (Viparita Karani).

This relaxed posture gives you an incredible feeling of calmness and relaxation all over your body and lets you take significant steps to develop your strength.

All you need is a wall!

How to bring legs up the wall?

- Begin by lying as more close as you could to the wall perpendicular to your left thigh.

- Lift up your legs and push them softly against the board.

- Seek to scoot so close as possible so that the knees against the wall are flat and the feet are stable.

- Relax your hands and put your arms on your sides straight.

- Hold your feet flexed and move your heels in.

- Taking steady inhalation and exhalation. It is a very soft stretch of the hamstring, and you can linger much longer anywhere between 5 and 10 minutes.

- Once the pose comes out, bend your knees or slip your legs off the wall and fall to your side.

Modification: When you notice your back hurt or can't straighten your legs, place a sheet or cushion under your sacrum for further comfort.

Ardha Parsvottanasana (Pyramid).

This pose is often referred to as Extreme Side Stretch, but don't let your name scare! It gives you a wide range, but you can tailor your yoga blocks to your tightness.

Where do I put Pyramid:

- Start from Mountain Pose and follow your left foot about 3,5 to 4 feet behind you. You just want to push up so much that both feet and both thighs can still be ground straight.

- Engage your knees and level your feet full. Then take an inhale and turn your upper body forward on the next exhale.

- You can either tie your hands behind the back with an extension of the shoulder, or you can use either side of the front foot for two supports. Set the block height depending on the tightness and use it to fold it deeper.

- In your hamstrings, you can feel a deep stretch, and your immediate instinct is to get rid of it. When this occurs, use your breath to return to the center and release any exhalation of tension and stress in the bee.

- On the other leg, repeat. One leg can be even closer than the other.

Change: Using a yoga block on either side is the perfect way to support yourself as you begin to deepen your position. Set the height according to the tightness and change slowly.

Halasana Plow Pose.

This posture is not only super successful in relaxing the hamstrings, but it also looks fantastic. You will not be able to reach the ground before you start running, but you will become more agile over time and will be able to do so!

Plow Pose How to Do:

- Begin with your flat feet on the floor on your back.

- Bring your legs, and your heels tucked towards your chest and put your hands on your shoulders.

- Straighten both knees to the wall and rotate both ankles.

- Begin to lower your feet over your head slowly and with purpose. Hold your hands for help on your lower back.

- Perhaps you can't lower your feet to the ground, but that's all right! Don't bend your knees enough to reach your toes, that's not going to stretch your hamstrings. You will hit the ground in no time of coaching.

- You will want to keep your hands under your lower back to feel more comfortable if you can never reach your feet to the floor or lift your arms to the level. It is always a fantastic turn of the elbow.

Change: Pose this in front of a wall and use the wall with your foot to continue and dig into the pose. It gives you more encouragement and power over the depth of your decision.

Facing Dog (Adho Mukha Svanasana) to the edge.

A man known knows what this posture is, you don't even do yoga. Yet its benefits are undoubtedly underrated!

It is a perfect strengthening and relaxing technique for the entire body, but it is particularly useful for those of you who want to enhance the flexibility in hamstrings.

You would definitely not be able to reach your foot as you launch first, so it will take you a while. You can see and hear a lot of change, be careful, and over time.

Why should I face down dog?

- Start all fours with your feet, dividing your inner hip-width, tucked toes, and hands directly under your arms.

- Move your hands up and down into the air on the next inhalation.

- Take the heart, shoulders, and legs into practice. Don't just let your body hang out in this place. You will know if you have all the weight on your shoulders that you are not spreading your weight correctly.

- Drag your feet in. You look like you are enjoying a fantastic stretch. Continue "pumping" the legs by stretching them one by one while warming them up.

- Keep totally committed to this role and really drive your heels all the way to get the best line.

Modification: If you are too inflexible to do a downward dog, consider using two supports under your hands to support it. You may even attempt to do it against a wall with your feet on the wall.

BACK

Most individuals get lower back problems because of a variety of causes. This may be that it has a fragile heart or actually does not relieve stress in small places. The following poses are perfect for stretching all parts of the back carefully.

Cat and Cow (Bitilasana and Marjaiasana).

Although they are two different poses, add them as one because, without the other, you cannot have one!

The fluid series that it produces to melt the spine is what makes Cat and Cow so sweet.

Where to Place Cat-Cow:

- You should start on all fours, tucking or untucking your feet. Make sure that your hands are behind your arms.

- Drop your belly with your inhale, arch your back, and smile up to the ceiling. It's a donkey.

- As you exhale, hollow out your belly along your neck and turn your back to look at the table. That is a mouse. It is a pet.

- Move through this process a couple of times and take the time to feel your body and any nearby places.

Modification: If it is too difficult to do this on your feet, seek a sitting cat-cow instead. Comfortable sit in a high position and step forward and loop your legs.

Camel Ustrasana

It is a perfect chest opener and a brilliant position to boost back agility. Cover yourself before undertaking this with a few cats and cows (position number 16) to avoid getting an unpleasant view in this position.

Camel Pose What to Do:

- Start with the rest of your body off the floor on your knees.

- Place your hands on your shoulders and start looking up and raise your face slowly. Naturally, you can begin forming a natural backbend with your body.

- Take your hands one at a time and keep moving across your mouth.

Modification: Use this pose with yoga blocks when you practice first. Place them at any height by your foot to build a milder backbend. You should work up slowly until you are able to do the entire thing. You should even keep your hands on your lower back to protect yourself, as seen above.

Spinal Bend Reclined (Supta Matsyendrasana).

Twists are excellent and soothing for the brain. There are so many different styles of contorted positions, but this is especially good for enhancing back strength and relieving tension.

Reclined Spinal Twist What to Do:

- Start with your knees and feet flat on the ground on your back.

- Place your elbows in your lap and place your right hand on your left leg on the ground.

- Begin lowering your legs slowly to the right and using your right hand to intensify the twist.

- Be sure your feet are kept on the ground and don't allow your legs to move right. This would lack the strength of the stretch.

- Extend your left arm straight across and cause your eyes to remain directly above the ceiling or to slip to the left.

- Move to the middle grade, then repeat on the other hand.

Position of the Infant (Balasana).

The pose of the child is mostly used as a rest during yoga sequences but also as a healthy posture to strengthen the stability of the spine. There are different variants, but the one that you will demonstrate is the easiest way to ease anxiety in the back.

How to do the pose of the child:

- Start on all fours on hip legs apart.

- Start to move your ass back on your heels slowly and let your forehead with your top body fall on the surface.

- Stretch your hands as far as you can by slowly pushing them out with every exhalation.

Change: If you want to stretch any further, try walking your hands on one side of your body and get a beautiful stretch to your leg. Do so at the exhalation, sit here for a few breaths, and then repeat for the other side.

Front Fold is standing (Uttanasana).

This is the last pose. This is the best way to relieve anxiety, improve strength, and stress and relax the body.

How to do Continuing Fold:

- Start at Pose Peak.

- Pick up your arms above, and then exhale your hands together and dive slowly down the middle until you hit bottom.

- They may even put their hands on their knees, then hinge slowly down, and then put their hands on the concrete.

- You can either put your hands on your shins, or you can use blocks to minimize the space on the floor, so you cannot reach the level.

- Make sure you hold straight in this place and lengthen your spine.

- You should even cover the foot with a brace and use the rope to fall a little deeper.

Change: You can use a brace or attempt to put two blocks at your feet to change the height to provide further protection. This pose has been loved, and they serve you well.

HAMSTRINGS

Whether you're an athlete, at a desk, or new to yoga, you're most definitely hamstrings. Implement poses so importantly to relieve tight hamstrings as tight hamstrings can cause another discomfort, such as lower back pain.

Simple legged forward sitting fold (Paschimottanasana).

Another folding forward sitting posture, but when you do this one, you'll look totally different. Mainly in your hamstrings, you can feel the pull.

How to do straight-legged forward sitting folding:

- Start in place of the staff and rotate both feet.

- Shift some added skin to the hand such that you lie squarely on the sits.
- Lift up your shoulders, spread your legs slowly to touch your knees, ankles or shins.

Change: a harness will be very helpful to get into the gap further and get the most gain. Place it around your foot and take the strap and move your hands on the rope to make the stretch longer.

The Wall of the Legs (Viparita Karani).

This relaxed posture gives you an incredible feeling of calmness and relaxation all over your body and lets you take significant steps to develop your strength.

All you need is a wall!

How to bring legs up the wall?

- Begin by lying as more close as you could to the wall perpendicular to your left thigh.

- Lift up your legs and push them softly against the board.

- Seek to scoot so close as possible so that the knees against the wall are flat and the feet are stable.

- Relax your hands and put your arms on your sides straight.

- Hold your feet flexed and move your heels in.

- Taking steady inhalation and exhalation. It is a very soft stretch of the hamstring, and you can linger much longer anywhere between 5 and 10 minutes.

- Once the pose comes out, bend your knees or slip your legs off the wall and fall to your side.

Modification: When you notice your back hurt or can't straighten your legs, place a sheet or cushion under your sacrum for further comfort.

Ardha Parsvottanasana (Pyramid).

This pose is often referred to as Extreme Side Stretch, but don't let your name scare! It gives you a wide range, but you can tailor your yoga blocks to your tightness.

Where do I put Pyramid:

- Start from Mountain Pose and follow your left foot about 3,5 to 4 feet behind you. You just want to push up so much that both feet and both thighs can still be ground straight.

- Engage your knees and level your feet full. Then take an inhale and turn your upper body forward on the next exhale.

- You can either tie your hands behind the back with an extension of the shoulder, or you can use either side of the front foot for two supports. Set the block height depending on the tightness and use it to fold it deeper.

- In your hamstrings, you can feel a deep stretch, and your immediate instinct is to get rid of it. When this occurs, use your breath to return to the center and release any exhalation of tension and stress in the bee.

- On the other leg, repeat. One leg can be even closer than the other.

Change: Using a yoga block on either side is the perfect way to support yourself as you begin to deepen your position. Set the height according to the tightness and change slowly.

Halasana Plow Pose.

This posture is not only super successful in relaxing the hamstrings, but it also looks fantastic. You will not be able to reach the ground before you start running, but you will become more agile over time and will be able to do so!

Plow Pose How to Do:

- Begin with your flat feet on the floor on your back.

- Bring your legs, and your heels tucked towards your chest and put your hands on your shoulders.

- Straighten both knees to the wall and rotate both ankles.

- Begin to lower your feet over your head slowly and with purpose. Hold your hands for help on your lower back.

- Perhaps you can't lower your feet to the ground, but that's all right! Don't bend your knees enough to reach your toes, that's not going to stretch your hamstrings. You will hit the ground in no time of coaching.

- You will want to keep your hands under your lower back to feel more comfortable if you can never reach your feet to the floor or lift your arms to the level. It is always a fantastic turn of the elbow.

Change: Pose this in front of a wall and use the wall with your foot to continue and dig into the pose. It gives you more encouragement and power over the depth of your decision.

Facing Dog (Adho Mukha Svanasana) to the edge.

A man known knows what this posture is, you don't even do yoga. Yet its benefits are undoubtedly underrated!

It is a perfect strengthening and relaxing technique for the entire body, but it is particularly useful for those of you who want to enhance the flexibility in hamstrings.

You would definitely not be able to reach your foot as you launch first, so it will take you a while. You can see and hear a lot of change, be careful, and over time.

Why should I face down dog?

- Start all fours with your feet, dividing your inner hip-width, tucked toes, and hands directly under your arms.

- Move your hands up and down into the air on the next inhalation.

- Take the heart, shoulders, and legs into practice. Don't just let your body hang out in this place. You will know if you have all the weight on your shoulders that you are not spreading your weight correctly.

- Drag your feet in. You look like you are enjoying a fantastic stretch. Continue "pumping" the legs by stretching them one by one while warming them up.

- Keep totally committed to this role and really drive your heels all the way to get the best line.

Modification: If you are too inflexible to do a downward dog, consider using two supports under your hands to support it. You may even attempt to do it against a wall with your feet on the wall.

BACK

Most individuals get lower back problems because of a variety of causes. This may be that it has a fragile heart or actually does not relieve stress in small places. The following poses are perfect for stretching all parts of the back carefully.

Cat and Cow (Bitilasana and Marjaiasana).

Although they are two different poses, add them as one because, without the other, you cannot have one!

The fluid series that it produces to melt the spine is what makes Cat and Cow so sweet.

Where to Place Cat-Cow:

- You should start on all fours, tucking or untucking your feet. Make sure that your hands are behind your arms.

- Drop your belly with your inhale, arch your back, and smile up to the ceiling. It's a donkey.

- As you exhale, hollow out your belly along your neck and turn your back to look at the table. That is a mouse. It is a pet.

- Move through this process a couple of times and take the time to feel your body and any nearby places.

Modification: If it is too difficult to do this on your feet, seek a sitting cat-cow instead. Comfortable sit in a high position and step forward and loop your legs.

Camel Ustrasana

It is a perfect chest opener and a brilliant position to boost back agility. Cover yourself before undertaking this with a few cats and cows (position number 16) to avoid getting an unpleasant view in this position.

Camel Pose What to Do:

- Start with the rest of your body off the floor on your knees.

- Place your hands on your shoulders and start looking up and raise your face slowly. Naturally, you can begin forming a natural backbend with your body.

- Take your hands one at a time and keep moving across your mouth.

Modification: Use this pose with yoga blocks when you practice first. Place them at any height by your foot to build a milder backbend. You should work up slowly until you are able to do the entire thing. You should even keep your hands on your lower back to protect yourself, as seen above.

Spinal Bend Reclined (Supta Matsyendrasana).

Twists are excellent and soothing for the brain. There are so many different styles of contorted positions, but this is especially good for enhancing back strength and relieving tension.

Reclined Spinal Twist What to Do:

- Start with your knees and feet flat on the ground on your back.

- Place your elbows in your lap and place your right hand on your left leg on the ground.

- Begin lowering your legs slowly to the right and using your right hand to intensify the twist.

- Be sure your feet are kept on the ground and don't allow your legs to move right. This would lack the strength of the stretch.

- Extend your left arm straight across and cause your eyes to remain directly above the ceiling or to slip to the left.

- Move to the middle grade, then repeat on the other hand.

Position of the Infant (Balasana).

The pose of the child is mostly used as a rest during yoga sequences but also as a healthy posture to strengthen the stability of the spine. There are different variants, but the one that you will demonstrate is the easiest way to ease anxiety in the back.

How to do the pose of the child:

- Start on all fours on hip legs apart.

- Start to move your ass back on your heels slowly and let your forehead with your top body fall on the surface.

- Stretch your hands as far as you can by slowly pushing them out with every exhalation.

Change: If you want to stretch any further, try walking your hands on one side of your body and get a beautiful stretch to your leg. Do so at the exhalation, sit here for a few breaths, and then repeat for the other side.

Front Fold is standing (Uttanasana).

This is the last pose. This is the best way to relieve anxiety, improve strength, and stress and relax the body.

How to do Continuing Fold:

- Start at Pose Peak.

- Pick up your arms above, and then exhale your hands together and dive slowly down the middle until you hit bottom.

- They may even put their hands on their knees, then hinge slowly down, and then put their hands on the concrete.

- You can either put your hands on your shins, or you can use blocks to minimize the space on the floor, so you cannot reach the level.

- Make sure you hold straight in this place and lengthen your spine.

- You should even cover the foot with a brace and use the rope to fall a little deeper.

Change: You can use a brace or attempt to put two blocks at your feet to change the height to provide further protection. This pose has been loved, and they serve you well.

Yoga To Lower Stress Level

Peace between mind and body.

Yoga enhances your ability to calm, focus, stabilize, and sleep. The time you spend doing yoga and meditation helps you to calm and ease your mind. You will learn to focus your physical and mental resources more efficiently, making your tasks more critical, imaginative, and productive. And you're more focused at the moment as you concentrate your attention on breathing and shifting your body in space. The way to making the best of a position is not only to focus on your muscles but also to your respiration.

Flexibility and strength of the body

Yoga will help strengthen the endurance and strength of the body. Yoga promotes harmony in your entire body, making you relaxed and flexible. When your heart strengthens and your endurance increases, your stance changes naturally. Yoga aims to correct and improve your posture so that you can relieve the backpressure, change the feel, and make your body appear more relaxed. When you draw on your routine every day, it will have several potential advantages to strengthen your form and reduce your tension. You'll continue to feel the difference. Indoors you should feel better (both mind and body). You will begin to understand that you didn't have many things that troubled you before. Your relationships will continue to change. All when you feel less stressed, more relaxed, and more flexible, your muscles are more robust.

Mindful meditation included yoga.

When working on the mat, the way you breathe is most significant. A gentle Yoga Class is a considerable Yoga Class that focuses on yoga relaxation. Yoga involves rotating the body and creating multiple poses while respiring slowly and slowly. Every class concludes with a peaceful pause, meditation, and pranayama. Restaurant yoga is a gentler yoga type that concentrates on muscle relaxing and relaxed breathing. Vinyasa yoga is a fluid yoga style where breath gestures are made. Regardless of how you exercise, focus on the breath is essential to make the most of yoga and meditation. This is the easiest way to calm down and clear your head of all the chaos inside and around you.

Your Breath Works.

The cobra pose opens your chest to allow more oxygen into your lungs. Lift your hips slowly as your legs are squarely on the floor and fire your chest with your muscles so that your body appears like a cobra rising. When it's too hard to lift up with your shoulders, put your elbows on the concrete. Continue to reflect on your breath as you do. The trick is to respire vigorously from the abdomen and get as much fresh air in the lungs as possible. It would be pushed in and out when you inhale and exhale if you were to place a palm on the heart. Enable your chest, neck, side, and rib cage to stretch as you breathe in the air. You can feel your stomach rising and flattening as you breathe in and out of your nose, increasing your breathing rate. Don't breathe too fast, or you can feel light-headed! Note, you're breathing under the order.

Built-up anxiety and pain release.

There are some stress management activities that can also help to reduce stress and anxiety. While all stress is not bad, the excellent weight will help you get things done, and reduced stress causes physical and emotional pain and injury. A long, gradual exhalation and a deep inhalation are an essential way to relieve pain and tension. Yoga is a perfect way to de-stress and raising fear, as you might already learn. Education is critical for alleviating pain, particularly though you don't want to do yoga. You will smile and also laugh during meditation, which also relieves tension. Anybody enjoying yoga?

The lower body and the circulation of blood

Throughout Bikram Yoga, the warm space encourages inflammation that helps to expel contaminants from the body and relax and stretch muscles to avoid injury. Water flushes your body's harmful toxins and leaves your brain alert. As the body relaxes, the intestines loosen and continue to release toxins and waste. Pranayama helps the entire body to oxygenate and to flush out cell toxins. Through supporting the body function more appropriately, Japanese Yoga helps avoid and repair chronic injuries. This can help alleviate tension for and for a while.

A Common Way to Tension Contract.

Yoga helps for a sense of calm and understanding when coping for physical and psychological effects. Yoga makes you lose weight, is stress-free, and allows you to reach specific goals. Many psychiatric problems can be routinely treated with yoga. Yoga breathing alone will help people with physical disabilities. Pain is a significant factor in aging and allows for quicker aging. The pain was also known to lead to many other diseases. Sounds of visual pictures of tension washed or brushed away, and you will be able to withstand everyday pressures and the burden on your mind and body better.

Least from 10 to 20 minutes a day.

A fast way to better relieve tension is to lay down and shut your eyes anytime you wake up for a few minutes. To order to perform pranayama, you might want to sit cross-legged or lay on your back so that you are comfortable. Relax at the end of the session and lay on your back 5-20 minutes with your eyes closed. You say ten to yourself with the first breath, and you say nine with the next breath, and so on. You will close your eyes and imagine yourself in your dream vacation destination. Usually, you spend between 5-10 minutes in intense meditation at the end of a yoga session, in particular, Hatha.

We may have our own way of dealing with pressures, so are we doing well? Yoga and meditation sessions regularly (at least many days a week) provide you with tools to help you handle the depression much better. You will learn and develop it as you continue to train. Namaste. Namaste.

The eternal art of yoga is still perfect for everything. Continue the Yoga practice through pregnancy as long as you pay careful attention to limits and body! Prenatal yoga is healthy enough to stay if you haven't already done yoga, but it is clearly better to train yourself before you get pregnant in a perfect future. The combinations and poses used in prenatal yoga are, however, flexible and appropriate for those who do or do not.

The body evolves drastically through birth, and Prenatal Yoga is a perfect way to calm down and enjoy what your body really feels. After all, there's a whole new guy!

Prenatal yoga brings your mind down and softens your breathing that is so important in moments of fear, tension, and unexpected issues.

Discuss your wish to perform prenatal Yoga with your doctor first, and all other forms of exercise during pregnancy, whether it be usually either once a week or more. All types of use during breastfeeding are advised to be monitored by physicians for your and the health of your infant.

Take it in the first trimester very quickly and softly. Stay until your pregnancy has ended until your exercise and workout plans begin or commence. Get yourself fit and relaxed with things like cycling, swimming, and soothing yoga that will help your pregnancy to stabilize and get healthy. When you become more energized in the second quarter, higher rates of operation will begin. The third quarter will again be quicker because you are much overweight and you're tired!

Prenatal yoga breathing is later than usual and is related to activity more often than not. Those deeper and longer breaths will fill the lungs so that you and your baby can fully gain precious oxygen and goodness. Deep breathing is a perfect way to relax the body and mind, even helpful when in the middle of a row or disaster and alleviate pain and anxiety. Total exhalation and relaxation lets help you to feel calmer, more confident, and more energetic later on.

Understanding how to practice this smoother and more relaxed way of breathing during prenatal yoga will help prepare you for life, conception, and a new baby. Breathing will allow you to stay comfortable, especially during workplace contractions, and will allow you to relax and let go.

Pregnant women have a quicker speed in yoga than usual. It is easy to get lost in the fact that you don't want to gain too much weight through pregnancy and want to keep fit at the same speed as before, but trust me, consider what your body does - it makes a little baby, and you gain a low weight or not. Creation structures it because you require extra pressure to support and nurture your infant!

It is essential, yes, to keep fit and healthy, just not so concerned with it! Talk to your body to stop being forced or stressed past what you need. For your child's creation, vital energies and goodness are required, not your ego!

Avoid poses that rest entirely on your stomach, especially in the 2nd and 3rd sections. Stop doing the Cobra in both front and abdominal positions!

Yoga during breastfeeding is a perfect way to spontaneously enhance the desire to deliver your infant. Listed positions and gestures are intended to help increase the baby's chance of getting into an ideal birth location.

When you are allergic, allergic, reviewed with your doctor, and have no excuse not to do prenatal yoga, three days a week is the absolute number of sessions to try and fit. What is important is that you listen and do what's best for your body and instincts!

We're both individuals, and no two women have the same body! Hear how you feel and how your body feels and then determine what you most wanted! On different days, you will feel different, so relax when you need it, and you will do yoga when you need it. Regardless, try to relax thoroughly and comfortably and to sustain energy levels by feeding and drinking plenty of water too!

Please take as many breaks as you like during your prenatal yoga session and rotate the more demanding and soothing positions. During the pregnancy, the Relaxin hormone is plentiful and can loosen the muscles and ligaments preparing to give birth. It is also indispensable not to expand it or push it into places.

When you are pregnant, lying on your back is still a problem. First of all, people rested on their backs for thousands of years without any issues; however, the reason it is not today is that the baby will not get into the ideal position or to get the best oxygen from the placenta, which lies on the left side. Lying on the left-hand side is strongly recommended for sleeping and resting, and after the 20th week of pregnancy, it is advised not to lay on the back.

Most women wake up, and that's all right, don't worry. When you lay under your knees on your bottom, the weight isn't so hard on your base. Lie on your left side if you have a preference.

Your bowels continue to appear and bulge in the second quarter (and note that all the bumps are different shapes and sizes), and you begin to feel your baby's movement. Massaging the belly is now necessary to help reduce stretch distances and help with elasticity.

You'll have more stamina during the second trimester, and you will want to do a lot more, particularly if you've had nausea in the first trimester! That is when prenatal yoga is done! Many women during this time feel vibrant and blooming, and prenatal yoga will allow you to feel even more fantastic.

For balance and coordination, firm standing stances and squatting with the ball help to loosen the hips and support a healthy conception! Much versatility is extraordinary to brace the hips for birth and helps to get the baby in the correct and desired birthplace!

Your belly will be high in your 3rd trimester! Prenatal Yoga in the third quarter helps you more relaxed. Your body keeps developing and relaxing (reassure you're massaging), and your baby's breathing is even more noticeable now.

You need to change your roles and places to match you! Between your feet, seats, bolsters, covers, and walls, you should use pillows. This will help to keep the lower back, legs, and core under control.

Prenatal yoga aims to reduce fluid accumulation and to clamp typically to women during the third quarter. Last but not least, yoga will change during pregnancy and position the baby accurately if not already. Any place will also transform babies.

It is important to remember that you should not squat if your baby is in breaks after 34 weeks, particularly!

The endless benefits include meeting new mothers, bonding, energy benefit, versatility benefit, relief from fatigue and tension, mobilizedness, infant contact, time out, pain and swelling reduction, helping to sleep, promoting improved birth posture, keeping health, feeling good and nausea.

Yoga Poses For The Strength

If you're a guy and want to develop power and endurance, here are a few poses you can take: forward plug. This pose lets you stretch hamstrings, thighs, and calves. The move also serves to support the legs.

To assume the position, you will stand with the hip-width of your feet and then fold softly to your knees and lower the torso to the table. Then hold out your legs to touch the floor or the ankles. You will keep this pose for one minute and move back to a standing posture if you feel anxiety build up.

The shifting lung manages to relax the tense thighs. This can be achieved by extending the groin, which supports the arms and legs.

To take action, you must start on your hands and knees and then walk between your hands on your right foot. You have to raise your back knee gradually by holding your right leg above your hip. Then put your back against the wall behind you and straighten your back leg.

If your spine is straightened, push your hips forward and bring the rear heel behind you. You will hold for one minute in this place.

This action strengthens back, neck, spine, and hip flexors.

You have to lie on the floor, your legs bent and your feet on the floor. You will then put your hands behind your ground and lean for support into your chest.

You should shift your legs at a 45-degree angle to the surface, while you strengthen your core muscles to hold your spine straight. Then move your hands and imagine you're pressing a book between your knees.

You will straighten your legs and hold your body straight as you rise through the sternum. You should click your feet's balls and stretch your toes wide.

Place the hands-on side of the thighs, holding the legs in line with the shoulders with your palms facing down. You will keep it for 30 seconds.

Here are some of the positions you can use to develop strength and versatility. To stop harm, you will go to a gym where you can exercise under the guidance of a professional trainer.

Active Yoga Chair Poses?

Traditional yoga poses make it look like only trained ballerinas and contortionists can do yoga, but do you know that you can produce the same effects with a chair?

And is it stealing

This is called chair meditation. Chair meditation.

Whether you like to use the word "fancier," it's a new type of traditional Hatha Yoga.

Therefore, it is time to develop confidence and improve equilibrium.

It is one of the main problems for the disabled due to accidents contributing to injury. Healthy posture and agility avoid this.

Anything you're going to learn will be done from your dining room chair.

The three yoga poses to do, reducing the chance of dropping.

1. The tree rises up and raises your head if you can. Go you! Save home! Now place the other hand on the chair to support you. Then lift one hip, lean on the knee, and rest your foot at the top of the other bone. And take the position.

That is the beauty of the yoga pose for any elderly person to seek.

When you maintain this role, you strengthen your focus, flexibility, and posture. Practice it daily, and the feet stay securely planted and adequately balanced.

2-Do you recall using a flashlight to create silhouettes on the wall—rabbits humping, birds soaring or large gigantic shapes of dinosaurs, scaring the bejeezus out of the house for everyone?

Imagine that you can do it and emulate a dancer by placing the body in this role.

It is one of the modified chair yoga movements and is performed without a chair in traditional yoga. Highly rough.

You lift your leg first with your hand on the same side to keep your foot behind you. The other side will go right in front of you. Because it is altered for the aged, using the chair to hold your weight as you stand on one knee and brace the other foot on the other hand.

The role of the dancer gives you a sense of beauty as you wear it, and it's incredible to lift your mind and to improve your stamina.

3-The Eagle Mind the silhouettes above. You're here to do so, except you won't pilot the shadow eagle.

You are sitting in the chair, cross the leg, and keep the spot. The motions should be made with the body. Place their arms in front of them and let them step over.

Then bring your forearms together in a vertical stance, where you press each other on the back of your hands.

The adult posture and arm movements are perfect for relaxing the shoulder muscles and assisting with breathing power.

CHAPTER FOUR

The Important Of Yoga Pose

The Emperor of Yogic Asanas is the Headstand or Shirsasana. Just put, an asana is a yogic pose or location of the body.

The torso is entirely twisted and held upright by the forearms while the head crown lies gently on the surface.

This reversal mechanism is what makes headstand so secure, mainly because it reverses the force of gravity. Force pushes us typically back and compresses our heads, but this cycle becomes totally reversed as we reverse. Instead, gravity works on us by decompressing our bodies and restoring circulatory and lymphatic system currents.

Which are the benefits of the booth?

Regardless of your yoga style or stage, reversals revitalize and rejuvenate the entire body. Turning your body upside down reverses gravity and nourishes your vital organ and brain. The pineal and hypophysial receptors are stimulated, and the hormones are regulated. The lifting of the legs increases the circulation, vein retention, and lymph drainage, which relieves pressure which exhaustion. Inversions also aid relax, eat, calm, and relaxed muscles.

Creating improvements and investing time back and forth every day is one of the best things you might do about yourself. Inversions are basically a vitality elixir.

Gravity slowly but inevitably weighs us down and diminishes our energy. We stand, sit, or walk upside down with our arms, legs, and pelvis below. As the years go by, so do the damage. Subcutaneous fat sags. Fat sags. Hemorrhoids and varicose veins erupt. The heart tired, weary of pumping blood continuously across the vast circulatory network. The ancient yogi called gravity the invisible adversary. The yogi carried out sleight of hand martial arts: rise up and use the strength of gravity to combat the ravage of the same self-force.

The human body is prone to gravity variations as it consists of about 60% fat. The body is porous from the surface of cells suspended in an intercellular fluid bowl. A dynamic vessel network weaves in and around all cells and transfers fluids continuously through pipes, pumps, and pore membranes to store, wash, feed, and purify liquids.

When you invert, the lower extremity of the skin fluids drains much more rapidly than when you sleep. Congestion zones open. If you will stay upright for only 3 to five minutes, the blood not only flows quickly into the heart, but tissue fluids circulate more effectively to the lower extremities and lymph channels of the abdominal and pelvic organs to promote a healthy nutrient and waste exchange between the cells and capillaries.

"Sirshasana(headstand) is a gift and nectar. Words do not sufficiently explain the positive outcomes and consequences. In that asana alone, the brain will absorb a lot of Prana and energy. Memory is developing admirably, and judges, occultists, and philosophers can genuinely enjoy the Asana. Investments are also calming and raising tension and pressure correctly. During Sirsasana, the supply of blood to the brain is increased, the exhausted cells are rejuvenated, and the mind is activated. It activates the pituitary and pineal glands that are dependent upon a person's development, health, and vital energy.

Nourishes pituitary and pineal glands and activates them. Headstand offers cleaned blood and waters, in particular, and nourishes the hypothalamus, pineal gland, and hypophysiology. Within the endocrine system, these drums play aa significant part. The endocrine system uses hormones to regulate cell metabolism. Our production, wellbeing, and longevity depend on how these two glands work correctly, which regulate the body's chemical balance. The secretions of the hypophysis control sexual property and the production of reproductive organs. The function of the adrenal, thyroid, and ovaries is also regulated. It is the hormone that increases milk production in mothers. The hypophysis is, therefore, the main gland that plays a crucial role in the regulation of menstruation and pregnancy. The inverted locations control the function of the master gland in order.

Inversion of the circulatory system stimulates the heart and facilitates venous reversal. Inversions do almost the same for the body as aerobics. "The central aspect for stretches of your cardiac muscle is the fluid transfer to the heart (vein reversal) and distension of the ventricles. Inversions require the advantage of gravity to get additional fluid into the heart-flipping yourself upside down facilitates vein reversal. This decreases heart pressure. Senile brain modifications are avoided. And as described before, ischemic strokes can be prevented absolutely, as the blood flows are improved without weight. "Call the brain to help alleviate discomfort to mild distress. It is vital, restful, and calming. A relaxing influence is felt on the face in the pose.

Yoga Poses For The Relaxation

Your time as a single mother is essential. Chair Yoga is a perfect way for busy mothers and women to work a quick yoga class into your hectic schedule.

The simple chair yoga can be practiced at home or at work anytime you feel drained, frazzled, and need a fast burst of strength in order to enjoy the day.

Which is Yoga Chair?

In short, Chair Yoga requires the focus of traditional yoga (asanas, breathing exercises, meditations, and relaxation), and you rest on the chair instead of standing or using a yoga mat. This makes Chair Yoga the perfect way to add yoga to your life, especially if you have little time and no desire to enjoy a full Yoga class.

Side notice: For all types of exercise, contact a doctor if you are suffering from chronic problems or back pain prior to this series. Try to show compassion and patience with your body during breathing exercises.

You can do yoga at your office, and you don't have to think about finding child care or leaving work, changing your wardrobe, and hurrying to a class.

The exercises help to relieve tension in the neck and shoulders and reduce regular pains and discomfort.

The routine refreshes your mind quickly and allows you to stay calm and concentrated, mainly when operating on a tight timeframe.

If you sense your motivation is fading as you want to concentrate on what you are meant to do, take a 5-minute break and do this secure chair yoga method, instead of wasting more time and resources. You'll feel energized, refreshed, refocused, and ready to resume work again.

Eight simple chair yoga exercises and fast energy boost, sit comfortably on your chair. Lengthen your back, raise your head so that your chin is in contact with your shoulders in a straight line. Relax your mouth, lower your return. Take a prolonged deep nasal intake and breathe out slowly. Repeat three to five times. First, flex and curl your toes and place your feet on the floor securely.

Remain in the position above, breathe in, and gently put your hands together in your arms. Close your head. Open your eyes. Inhale quickly into a count of three and exhale steadily into a count of three. Attempt three or five times three. Hold the hands touching; raise your arms in the air above your head slowly. Hold your head straight and loosen your jaw. Keep your head tilted and give a relaxed look straight ahead. Take three to five rounds of deep breaths as you stretch your body edges.

Stretch your arms to the right / left Next, tie your fingers, loosen your index fingers, and point up. Hold your chair seated, stretch your body to the right, and keep your head parallel to the table. Seek to keep the knees and shoulders in a straight line. Take three deeper breaths and then go back to the middle. If your arms are tired, turn your hands back into your lap and let your breathing relax. Repeat gradually, stretching this time to the west. Take 3-5 deep breaths and head back to the center.

Place your palms on your knees, seated Cobra. Take note that your feet are still flat on the ground going forward. Respire in and out, raise the chin, drop the head back, and backward. Keep your head bowed and loosen your jaw. Breathe in and breathe out slowly. Repeat three to five times. Transfer the body to the core gradually.

Place your hands on your knees, raise the arm up to the point of the shoulder. Make a fist and turn your arm in each direction 5-7 times. Then open your fist for 30 seconds and softly shake your palms. Put your hands on your lap. Hold hands.

Place your body so that your feet are squarely on the surface, lengthen your spine, and loosen your neck. Seated spinal twist Pass over your right hip with your left leg. Place your right hand on your leg bent. Keep your back straight. Turn your spine slowly towards the left, looking over your left side. Keep your back straight and comfortable while you breathe three or five rounds deep. Coming back to the middle grade. Uncross your hands. Uncross your hands. Place your left hand on a bent knee and slowly tilt your body and look on your right shoulder. Test your foot and body lines properly. Finally, lift your back when you look over your right shoulder. Take 3-5 deep breaths and head straight to the middle.

Concentrate on your breath, place your hands on your chest, face-up, straighten your spine, shut your eyes and enjoy the last few moments your place and the sensations and emotions that run through your body.

When you're ready, open your eyes slowly, smile, and embrace.

HEALTH BENEFITS OF YOGA

Yoga, which derives from the Sanskrit word "Yug" means linking, combining, combining, and yoking. This usually translates to the union of body, mind, and soul in its practice. Yoga provides a tremendous wellness advantage in this holistic approach to well-being.

Yoga offers positions or asanas which can work for any bone, muscle, ligament, and tendon in the body. Such apparently different postures work together in the right order and under professional direction in unison to deeply massage all the internal organs of the body. This relaxation and organ massage holds illness away and also warns of the imminent onset of the disorder.

HEART.

According to recent studies from the Medical School of Yale University, yoga will improve the heart's health in just six weeks, for an hour and a half, three days a week. Diverse positions of yoga and controlled breathing techniques increase the absorption of oxygen in the blood in a shorter time. It means that the cardiovascular muscles receive healthy oxygen, which helps prevent coronary artery disease and preserves the overall health of the heart. Sustained yoga also decreases cholesterol by the increased blood supply and fat burning.

Mountains, warriors, triangles, trees and lotus poses are excellent for the heart. Kapaalbhati's controlled breathing technique also helps to keep the heart-healthy.

SYSTEM VENTILATION.

Structured breathing techniques like nasal alternations, help clear the nasal passages that reduce signs of sinusitis and allergy. Yoga also stresses proper and full breathing and uses the entire upper body to do so. Therefore, tightness around the arms, back, chest, and abdomen can impede the ability to take a full breath. Yoga postures broaden these areas to reinforce them to promote deep breathing. This which the respiratory rate, which shows that the lungs function better.

Asanas are raised knees, ladder, chair, cobra, and mountain positions rather than breathing exercises that aim to expand the chest cavity.

Spin and Center Systems.

The muscle portions of the previous ones are reversed by following asanas in a healthy yoga routine. Yoga uses free weight, i.e., for strength training, your own body weight. These two things improve backbone strength and ensure excellent overall spinal safety. Yoga decreases spine compression and helps minimize back pain and body balance. In fact, the ability of yoga to lower cortisol levels helps maintain calcium in bones, reduce the risk of osteoporosis.

Pills and cobra pose used to reduce lower back pain. For optimal half plow, spinal safety, axle, bow, spinal twist, and mountain positions are advised. For a fact, the standing wheel posture is used to remedy slight scoliosis or spinal curve. Yoga has a specific category of attitudes, such as the Bramha pose, which is primarily intended to strengthen and relax the neck muscles, which is typically ignored in other types of yoga.

Yoga activates the parasympathetic nervous system, lowering blood pressure and easing the breath to calm. Faced with dog's downstream, back, shoulder braces, bridge, and half-moon pose, discomfort from sciatica may be reduced. Recent research reveals that yoga can lead to rising brain gamma-aminobutyric rates (GABA). The development of Alzheimer's is associated with higher GABA levels. Focusing on stress reduction, respiration, and restoration of the overall body balance can help prevent epileptic seizures.

SYSTEM LYMPHATIC.

Yoga focuses on the usually disregarded muscles and body parts and helps the lymphatic system to act. Headstands, spinal twists, and reversals tend to eliminate contaminants and expel substantial lymph across the chest.

ORGANS ABDOMINAL.

Sustained yoga practice encourages improved posture to improve the efficiency of the digestive and disposal processes. This not only improves the digestive tract's blood supply but also enhances bowel activity to boost the digestion. The relaxing effect of yoga relaxes the nervous tract and helps to expel stored toxins more efficiently.

Many asanas enhance blood supply to the hepatic cells, sensitize lymph nodes, and strip away contaminants from the peritoneum and hepatic regions. Good liver leads to cholesterol loss, improved absorption, and better blood metabolism. Yoga helps your muscles remove excess glucose from the blood of the body and makes it more useful for the pancreas and liver to function. It also allows the pancreas to produce more insulin and will raise blood sugar levels. Because a healthy yoga regimen stretches every muscle in your body, it holds your entire body fit. Yoga is particularly helpful for diabetic patients with these conditions.

For abdominal regions, it is advised to have Kapalbhatti, spinal twists and half plough, ships, raised knee, the lock of hands, and bolt poses of thunder.

Kids.

Many yoga poses, like the warrior pose, are highly useful for the kidneys because they stretch your lower belly, activate your big bowels, avoid constipation, and increase urination. Specific asanas ideal for the kidneys and urinary tracts are pieces, vessels, plates, rising, and squat positions. Breathing Kapalbhatti due to its significant detoxifying effect helps to control the organs.

Head.

Yoga functions not only the body but the mind. As much of yoga is organized and maintains a pose, yoga practice encourages you to look inward and involves bright focus. It helps to manage a wandering mind that increases understanding of oneself and acceptance. The positive image of the self thus fights against depression. Controlled workouts and meditation will relax the mind. Better brain blood supply combined with decreased discomfort and higher concentration contributes to improved recall.

Deep breathing in a headstand increases the blood flow to the brain and stimulates the hypophysis that helps relieve mild depression. For outstanding mental well-being, other asanas recommended include the bridge, leg, guerrilla, palm tree, and childhood poses.

Some Divine Blessings.

Arthritis-The gradual and deliberate practice of yoga tends to alleviate the effects of arthritis. Because of the profound impact of yoga postures, moderate pressure on the joints is exerted, and the risk of damage is considerably reduced than in other types of exercise.

Cancer–Yoga has been found to increase the body's red blood cells. This helps cancer patients to fight chemotherapy anemia, nausea, and fatigue.

Migraine-Rhythmic breathing techniques tend to relieve attacks of migraine.

Cramps-Some yoga poses to stretch and relax the vaginal muscles. Squat and raise are particularly useful to reduce menstrual cramps and control cycles.

While yoga has many health advantages, real importance lies in its quality of life. You can gain greater control of your mind and body through continuous yoga practice. This sense of absolute joy is the total wellbeing reward of a yogi.

Yoga - Best For Body, Mind, and Spirit Wellness

Over the last century, we have discovered that our intellectual, physical, emotional, or spiritual nature is a part of our own being. This will redound to the detriment of the other component, for example, because one element, the emotional, is influenced adversely.

Nobody really accepts the risk of any health problems. The question is so true-to be or to restore health and stay fit? Most people started to talk about potential, practical, and efficient ways of doing it. Pain reduction and relief must be secure and reliable.

Yoga may be the solution to these questions.

The philosophy of Yoga centers on these three fundamental issues about body functions, including sleep, and techniques about breathing. Originating from the North, Yoga is now embraced and carried out in local and global cultures, as one of the ancient practices. His adherents started with religious organizations and now comprise businesses, specialist bodies, and ordinary civilians. This is now commonly known as how depression affects work efficiency and disrupts peace in a household and how yoga helps to relieve tension or relaxation.

Yoga looks at things in their entirety. Yoga emphasizes peace-bringing, body, mind, and spirit together. This idea helps you with tension, physical wellbeing, social consciousness, and spiritual change.

Yoga shows you how to meditate successfully, how to relax, imagine, flex your body, and gestures. Yoga poses stretch your spine as you learn to control and slow down your respiration. The body is relaxed and energized similarly.

If you stick to practicing yoga over time, you can avoid stress later. The full breathing routine, body exercises, workout schedules, meditation, and guided imagination alleviate the tension you now face.

Yoga also lowers blood pressure and adjusts heart rate, increases anxiety rates and muscle constriction, improves strength levels and limbs of the body.

Compared to the regular exercise sessions, yoga steps are gradual and gentle, which makes yoga accessible even to those who are physically affected by illness. Moreover, meditation and Yoga positions grow the mind and spiritual consciousness.

There's nothing good about dropping into our laps. You need to spend daily time for yourself before you can achieve those benefits which contribute to the health of your entire body. In time, you will soon know that joining yoga was the best decision you have ever made in your life.

Practice Yoga to Nourish Your Body and Your Soul

A heart that functions are typically a stress-free heart. Although that is often impossible to do in our running culture, there are also ways to tackle the relentless tension that we frequently face. Yoga has proven to be perhaps the most powerful method for overcoming the fear in our lives, and particularly in our minds and bodies.

Yoga will perform well for blood circulation, in particular. The external cardiovascular system is extended and relaxed at standing poses in order to allow a proper blood supply into the surrounding regions. The lymphatic pathway, attached to legs and arms, will direct the circulation further upward. The upper body is calm, regenerated, and ventilated in horizontal postures, which helps reduce blood pressure levels. Last but not least, when plied attentively and without pressure, the blood inside the myocardium can quickly improve to the tones of the heart muscle.

Yoga exercises are also aerobic in nature based on how easily a person takes the pose. The greeting of the sun is an outstanding example. If this mixture of locations is appropriately done, pumping starts in the heart to improve blood supply. The perfect method for relaxing the mind and reducing fear significantly decreases the movement in these places.

The Sun's Salutation: Begin with the hands pressed and fixed to the heart in the mountain. Taking a deep breath and hold your hands above your head while leaning over. Exhale gently as you lay your hands away. Cover the upper portion of the body to a lateral yet upward curve.

Inhale as you push your right leg into a chest. Breathe out and straight to Plank Positioning, position the left knee. Maintain this place and breathe in. Respire out and drop the body to the ground. Thrust the upper body during inhalation and raise the hands like an Upward Dog. Switch to Downward Dog by extending the knees and lifting the legs.

Move the left foot to the Lunge with an inhalation. Respire and switch the right leg to Standing Forward Bend. Raise your upper body as you relax and raise your arms above your head so that you have a slight backbend in your posture.

Finally, after the exhalation, place your hands down and return to the first position, the Stance, with palms attached to the face. Repeat the routine on the other side to complete the whole series. If you finish five rounds, you do a perfect method early in the morning.

Lower Blood Pressure Research has found that daily yoga slows one's pulse rate, stimulates healthy blood flow, and decreases blood pressure rates. Volunteers who took a yoga course for six weeks were reported to increase their circulation (pattern of arteries contracting and relaxing to promote blood circulation) by 17%. Participants of cardiovascular disease have reported a 70% increase.

Most Asanas have a calming effect on the human body that decreases blood pressure and metabolism. Postures that involve long breathing rhythms significantly lower the body temperature. Perform the following positions to reduce elevated blood pressure levels.

Place of the legs up the wall: go to the wall and curl up to the bone. Then lean back and rest your legs on the ground. Hold the legs very straight and retain them vertically. Shift the foot and weight of the abdomen from the knees into the upper body. Relax and move your eyes until you see your face. If you sense a pull, step away from the wall slightly. Smoothly and thoroughly inhale from 5 to 10 minutes.

Some asanas are especially useful to alleviate anxiety. When you suffer an assault of fear, switch to bridge and plow positions. The Bridge relaxes the mind and lifts the lungs and refreshes sore thighs and legs at the same time. The Plough allows the endocrine system to stabilize while repairing the central nervous system. It is possible to reduce anger and relieve depression.

The Bridge Pose: lie on your back with your foot planting next to your fetus and palm trees. Inhale, drive the heels into the mat in order to raise the butt bone. Clamp the palms firmly and cover the shoulder blades, so the body weight rests on the triceps and feet. Low your hands. Lift your thighs. Wait for several breaths and roll down the vertebras slowly, one vertebra each time.

The Plough Position: Lie your back again with your hands to the side and straighten the legs to the left, put your feet, and stiffen your knees. Support the legs on an exhale and raise the hips to the chest. Remove the shoulder blades from the head and extend the upper body. On another step, move the lower back and legs upward with the hands and stretch the legs above your shoulders, putting the feet on the surface. Hold the thighs involved by bending the knees to fit between the neck and the legs. Inhale and exhale slowly and take as long as it sounds good. Move down one vertebra every time to relax. Relax on the back flat for a couple of deep breaths.

A normal inhalation and exhalation rhythm is a vital factor for minimizing tension and sustaining a healthy heart. The yoga or Pranayama has a curious power to relax and stimulate an exhausted body, a nervous heart, or a mad mind. For the next exercise, make an effort to distribute the respiration through your lungs equally.

The seated meditation: just quietly close your eyes. Tune your breath, be careful of the average circulation in your nose. When thoughts drift, only return the mind to the air. Begin with five minutes a day and slowly can as long as possible. The wind is a calm mind's anchor. Through constantly reminding the intention to stay still and concentrate on an event or thought, such as the rising and dropping tide, anxiety is removed from the emotional mind and allows physical and psychological stimulation.

Nadi Shodana is known to reconcile the two main energy flows (nadis) of the energy corpus (pranayama kosha), which are more or less like the extroverted and introverted parts of our individual. It further combines the left and right intellectual hemispheres and increases the flexibility of thought. Live in a comfortable position. Place the right hand in front of the face as you fold the index and middle fingers internally. Place the thumb next to the chin, and the ring finger next to the left cheek. Cover your right nose thumb and inhale steadily but deeply from your mouth. Then wait. Wait. Cut your right nose and replicate the same on the opposite side of your mouth. When done, slowly but totally exhale. This was Nadi Shodana's complete round. Start with 5 to 10 rounds and increasing the amount as the comfort and ease levels improve.

Daily yoga exercises remarkably activate, relaxes, and tones the skin. You should enjoy your body for Asanas as part of your everyday routine.

CHAPTER FIVE

Yoga Essential Needs For Health Benefits

Yoga is the ideal type of fitness for many healthy citizens. It is a healing program that strengthens the body, concentrates the mind, and helps to build a sense of spirit. Yoga is an ancient philosophy and fitness system that encourages unity between mind, body, and spirit. The term yoga is derived initially from the Sanskrit term "yoke" or "together." Yoga strives primarily to create a sense of peace and equilibrium between mind and body.

Yoga is the only discipline that allows one to introvert both body and mind, to emerge new. Yoga is an instructional program that is moral, emotional, and physical for people of all ages. It calms the spirit, improves focus and mental awareness, and thus reduces tension and anxiety. A real yoga practitioner seeks to cultivate a relaxed mindset. Health is a sacred gift granted by God. We will also preserve it not only to accomplish earthly ends but to represent the divine.

The aim of Yoga Yoga is to strengthen and stretch the body and to awaken the spirit–to maintain physical, mental, and spiritual health network. Yoga improves flexibility, raises oxygen absorption, and enhances the function of aerobic, metabolic, endocrine, reproductive, and disposal processes. This is achieved through physical exercises (asanas), relaxation techniques, and meditation. Yoga is soothing as it requires the mind and spirit.

Yoga can help reduce blood pressure and increase lung performance. People of all ages can do yoga; nearly all, including the elderly, babies, pregnant women, and people with chronic health conditions, will benefit from yoga. There is also a considerable body of evidence that yoga will support a variety of disorders, such as high blood pressure and diabetes. Obesity is typically one source of diabetes. Diabetes and obesity are sometimes called twin epidemics. Obesity and diabetes are also strongly preventable by adequate diet, exercise, and improvements in lifestyle. Yoga Lifestyle is ideally geared to handling this second outbreak. Yoga is difficult to "heal" diabetes, it can complement the dietary changes required in order to control diabetic symptoms, and it can make you feel more in control of your health and well-being. Today's life is full of stress and pressure, anxiety and nerve pain, excitement, and urgency. When man placed the simple concepts of Yoga into practice, he would be much more able to deal with his active life.

Yoga gives beauty, harmony, and lasting good fortune. You will also get calmness in mind when doing yoga. You should relax in peace. You can improve your strength, vigor, stamina, durability, and wellness. Within a limited time, you can do productive work. With any way of life, you will excel. Yoga will instill new strength, trust, and self-confidence in you. Body and mind are at your disposal. The body is God's temple. It is also our responsibility to keep it safe, healthy, and fragrant by cultivating compassion and caring.

Yoga gives you the courage to face the struggles of life. Likewise, you prefer to do activities that improve your strength by loving your body. Most yoga students are vegetarians and adopt a macrobiotic diet. In comparison to other workouts, yoga is more effective. It's not like we have to practice yoga every day or try to attend a yoga class once a week.

Yoga is widely recommended for those in a busy, demanding work environment, those with headaches, back or knees, allergies, and asthma, especially for those over 40 years of age (though younger, the better) Yoga is heavily suggested.

Yoga allows people to feel calmer and more confident and emotionally alert and healthy. Although yoga is an excellent type of self-help therapy, it is recommended to begin with a course taught by a trained instructor. There are several illustrated books on the subject, but nothing stops you from practicing yoga at home. Nonetheless, as a novice, you can gain even more from attending a college.

You shouldn't do things that your body isn't ready for before you get going. No head sits, bends backward, or pushes you into a cross-legged stance. A standard beginner class focuses on relaxing back, knees, and shoulders and consists of five to six standing positions, few floor positions, rest, and breathing at the end. Deep breathing is an aspect of Yoga practice that helps to make the body more alkaline.

A good class should have a structure: the instructor should clarify a situation and then come to rectify it if you're incorrect. You will feel healthy, whole, and stretched when you go out of the lesson and never tired.

Yoga courses can be held in towns and communities around the world. Very little equipment is needed, and a yoga session can be successful only for short sessions. However, it is more helpful if you can do 30 to an hour of daily sessions. Sessions will be conducted either in the morning or in the evening. Enable three hours to relax before doing yoga after a meal. Do not take a bath or shower half an hour before or during exercise.

Throughout the practice, you have to learn how to relax after an operation. Citizens spend about a third of their time resting, attempting to regain their strength and health throughout the day. Great relaxation for the "real" form of relaxation is sometimes misunderstood. Also, calming music is noise when we are quiet. Yoga practitioners should observe the absolute quiet. Natural lovers are more prone to silence, and this characteristic must be established from childhood. Yet most people find comfort and peace of mind in clubs and bars can be achieved today. After what they see as a long workday, people drink and finally kill them. Sadly, others have never done so because they have not mastered the fundamentals of calming. This can be done by yoga.

So Yoga is a beautiful way to get to know your body better, whatever your sex, yoga will change your lifestyle. Yoga is not a faith, and it is a practice. The potentials of union with a "profound ego" are enticing to others, and a profound turnoff to others. Using as many you like, so continue to train.

Yoga Benefits and Fitness

Yoga shows us how to keep the peace between multiple powers that work on our bodies. If we don't care about our bodies, yoga will teach us how to regain our wellbeing by taking charge of our minds and bodies. This is in our power to take responsibility for our bodies. There are certain fundamentals of yoga which should be practiced during yoga practice.

Practice frequently. Do yoga daily, including though you perform a few asanas or pranayama in one day. You will then determine how much time to devote to yoga every day and then observe it strictly. Beginners need not make really optimistic plans because yoga needs to be careful. Set and accomplish achievable goals; it gives encouragement to pursue the practice of yoga. Thirty minutes to an hour of yoga practice is suitable for beginners. Don't wait for miracles overnight. Do not struggle as you do asanas. Your success in yoga will depend on the beginning of yoga on your age and fitness. To most beginners, a month of yoga practice will produce good effects. In a clean and well-ventilated space, practice yoga by putting a yoga mat on the ground. When the environment is hot, yoga can be a beautiful activity in a lawn early in the morning.

Yoga workout session. It is advised that you have a set time for yoga practice every day. One to two hours before sunrise is the perfect time to perform yoga because the amount of oxygen is high, and disturbances are not present. If you see fit, yoga can even be done in the evening if you're not too sleepy. Before yoga, eat nothing three hours.

Ensure an appropriate diet. Ensure sure your food contains plenty of nuts, berries, salads, and leafy vegetables. Chew the meal properly. Don't rush when you eat fruit. If necessary, skip tea or coffee. Contain up to two cups of tea or coffee each day. Reduce the intake of calories, stop junk food, and fresh snacks. Strictly stop nicotine as it cancels the benefits of pranayama. Seek to avoid drinking. You need to change your diet slowly to make it a way of life.

Stop stubbornness. Constipation is one of the issues that can hinder you from thoroughly learning from yoga. Drink enough water and have enough nutrients in your diet to avoid illness. In the morning before the yoga session, the bowels will be open.

Mental frame in yoga thinking. Seek to always keep your mind clear and peaceful. Yoga is not complete because the brain starts to drift. In the most part, focus on the body part of the asana or on the breathing. For total health, strength, and stamina, a calm mind is necessary.

Yoga exercise generally includes the following aspects:

- Restricting feeling. Restricting senses.

- After a natural diet.

- Mind control. Ego control.

- Appropriate respiration and relaxation.

- Exercise daily.

- Daily meditation.

Continuous introspection to find self-improvement shortcomings.

Don't forget to relax for 5 to 10 minutes in shava asana after your yoga session.

YOGA AND DIET FOR PROSTATE HEALTH

A bloke thing is the Prostate Gland. This is one of the components of the body's urinary and reproductive system. It is a male gland composed of a number of smaller organs covering the urethra and part of the bladder. Fellas will be taken care of.

The enigmatic gland is tiny, doughnut-formed, at the base of the bladder. This causes people more grief than any other aspect of their organs, and prostate cancer will soon be Australia's top killer of people. While about 50% of Australian men may have some sort of prostate problem at any stage in their life, people never give their prostate a second thought-not a smart idea.

The essential purpose is to secrete an alkaline substance that is part of the sperm when the ejaculation occurs. The fluid feeds and provides sperm volume, along with other seminal fluids.

Walnut sized in young men, and prostate enlargement is typical in men over 50 and about 4 in 10 men over 60 years of age. Expansion happens as the urethra thickening of the urethra and the connective tissues block urinary flow.

Causes of prostate enlargement

- Aging. When the body gets older, innocuous nodules form in the prostate tissues that collect and swell the gland slowly. Eventually, the kidney is large enough to' press' or' strangle' the urethra to obstruct urination.

- High zinc levels. The prostate tissues typically have high zinc levels. Zinc rates decline slowly as you grow older.

- More than 50 testosterone levels begin to decrease. This raises the amount of dihydrotestosterone (DHT) that overproduces prostate cells.

- Postural deficiencies and obesity can also affect the health of the prostate. A bulky body and prolonged sitting periods bring more pressure on the pelvic area and perineum, leading to swelling in and around the prostate.

- Constipation may be a cause, too. Hardened feces and a rectum that is bloated create undue pressure on the prostate gland.

Prostate symptoms issue

- The simple point is that it is impossible to pass water. It is how the urethra is compressed by the penis blocking the wind. You can struggle or wait a bit before you can go.

- A slow urinary flow ends and then ceases. The river is smaller and less reliable.

- Unintentional discharge–a propensity to dribble urine may be close to incontinence.

- When it has begun, you may find it challenging to avoid urination.

- You use the toilet more often. There may be regular urination or urination to urinate 2 to three times during the night and during the day.

- Just after passing urine, you still get the sensation of incomplete bladder emptying.

- The thin veins in the bladder and urethra extend due to excessive obstruction. If you urinate, the veins may burst, and blood may fall into the urine. It can lead to excessive urination, termed dysuria.

- Lower arms, back, and legs, and sometimes impotence, can include moderate discomfort.

In general, the signs of people with weak pelvic floor muscles are very close. Both represent a weakness of the genital tissues, bladder and reproductive organs, and weakness of the perineum or Root Chakra or Mulabhanda.

Diet and vitamins help

Trace mineral zinc is essential to the maintenance of prostate health. In the prostate gland and male hormone activity, zinc is necessary. It is known as "male mineral," and requires sperm and seminal fluid to be created. Impotence and infertility may result from a deficiency.

It is now well known that prostate health has a link to the zinc content of prostate tissue.

Dietary advice

- Keep a low-fat diet and watch the levels of cholesterol.

- Include Omega-6 and Omega-3, which help regulate the function of the nervous system.

- Stir-fried, Baked, Steamed, or render salads rather than deep-fried.

- Consider low-fat over full-fat milk, and, if possible, make it vegan.

- Avoid dressings with creamy salad and creamy sauces that stir the heart and the liver.

- drink eight glasses of water a day–green tea is healthy for the prostate as well.

- Increase your fibrous, fresh vegetables and fruit daily intake, particularly in red and red-orange foods and increase your flaxseed oils, vitamins A, C, E B6, and cod liver oils.

- Test if your consumption of Vitamin D is sufficient, including sunset time, and encourage your mind to respond with music, exercise, or power naps to relieve your tension. Stress contributes immensely to imbalances at all stages of life (body, mind, emotion, and spirit).

- Avoid spicy foods (these are considered' rajasic' in yogic Ayurvedic terms) that can increase body heat, inner fire, and emotions.

- Seeds of watermelon have inherent diuretic properties that avoid excess urinary buildup.

- Stop or limit the consumption of alcohol. Seek not to drink for a few days, then reintroduce. Within a day, you should know that it helps or hurts the urinary effects. It is because alcohol affects the neck of the bladder and inhibits urination and can lead to agitated body and mind.

- Avoid decongestants and antihistamines which modify the natural process of removal of the body.

- Stop smoky conditions and indoor settings. There is ample evidence that tobacco smoking has significant impacts on the scale of the expanding penis, as do all the other adverse health consequences. It could be as blood vessels in the body influence how much oxygen and nutrient-rich blood flow through the liver and extremities.

- Avoid cocoa, cookie, tea, and chocolate soft beverages. Many people find their prostate issues with caffeine are exacerbated by a rise in caffeine in the neck of the bladder. Use the removal strategy again.

- Use zinc in the diet: it is known that zinc increases urinary symptoms and reduces prostatic scale, and therefore is efficient in avoiding and restoring prostate enlargement. Zinc-high vegetables include dried boobs, chalk, garbanzos, lentils, black-eyed tomatoes, beets, tomatoes, and whole grains. Oats, Pumpkin seeds, whole wheat, and rye are also available.

Use selenium, Evening primrose oils, and amino acids every day to sustain the role of a healthy cardiovascular and nervous system-especially glutamine, alanine, and lysine.

Why Yoga Can Assist — Yoga integrates all processes and resources in the body, increases the consistency of blood, metabolism, controls hormone development and release, digestion, and elimination, and helps to stabilize and relax minds and emotions. Yoga will simultaneously improve, release, and support and offer men the mental challenges needed according to the sequences, stamina, and concentration. Bad circulation can exacerbate prostate problems. Daily practice of yoga will improve the flow of blood, intensify the respiration and loosen neuropathic knots into the tone and feed all cells, muscles, joints, and tissue. Some congestion or diverted prana or chi or energy will then be released to restore well-being, and hence we will feel more connected with nature.

Yoga also tends to make people more relaxed rather than agitate their structures. It is particularly useful as it encourages people to relate to their vulnerable side

and discuss facets of their emotions, which they would
not usually do in strength aerobics or boxing lessons
without losing or subjugating their masculinity!
Women can learn to understand and respect their
own voice by sitting on the mat. Maybe they can also
start discovering perhaps sharing what is in them
more often.

Yoga is about building harmony in the soul, emotion,
and soul-the physical advantage is just a bonus. Asana
(postures) is what we do to relax and meditate with a
still, undistracted mind. It doesn't matter how much
longer you have a place than the person next to you–
which men particularly seem to overlook if the
competing voices and pride bark loudly in their ears!

Through having the perineal or root lock or base
chakra conscious, which regulates impulses, behavior,
confidence, and purity of blood, prostate symptoms,
and the sensation of feeling that is not helped, may be
alleviated. When you have been awake, you must then
work through the Base Chakra to reinforce and
regulate energy, which will restore power through the
spine and allow people to claim their manhood in a
secure, but peaceful manner.

There are perfect yoga positions (safe for beginners) to boost prostate safety-

- Baddha Konasana-enhances the flow of blood to the pelvis, lungs, prostate and bladder and boosts consciousness and strength to the Mulabhanda or Root Lock;

Sit upright together on a mattress with the foot with soles, legs apart. Place your fingertips along the outer edge of your feet, concentrate on lengthening your neck and lifting your shoulders with every inhalation, and lower back and tailbone on every expiry. Do against a support wall if it's complicated. Draw the strength (a small area between anus and genitals) when you breathe in contact with Mulabhanda. Engage the belly gently and extend the neck to relax and purify the digestive and reproductive organs.

- Adho Mukha Svanasana-strengthens, the arms, and legs, extend the spine, expands the chest and lungs, and strengthens the back. An excellent all-round picture!

Begin all the fours, hands under the shoulders with extended arms, elbows under the legs, feet underneath. When your breast falls down into your hips, exhale and raise buttocks while your legs straighten. The spine is loose, hands in line with the top shoulders, and knees bent while hamstrings are tense and the back lower straight. Keep and relax, as you grip your palms tightly and raise kneecaps into knees while lowering the heels to the floor. No facial stress. Hold the abdominals involved and stretch over the arms, shifting the armpits to each other. Relax in childhood stance, head to floor, arms by your chest, and heels for a couple of breaths.

- Bhujangasana, knees bent up to the ceiling with their palms, touches the kidneys even more intensely and assists control the hormonal surge. It also helps to improve the development of all-male hormonal fluids by stimulating specifically the heart, organs, and sexual glands.

Lay your ass, palms with fingers spread out above your face, forehead down. Beats hip-width apart, continue grinding into the mat the pubic bone and the ends of your legs and feet and pulling the shoulders from your hands and elbows toward each other. Inhale and gently pull off a mat, keeping your arms around the ribs and stretching your elbows and shoulders. Keep it relaxed and press pubic bones, naves, and legs tightly into the mat for a few breaths. Don't get up too high it jams or straightens your wings. Look at the floor, so the neck remains high and stretches the chest and lungs from the pubic bone to the head, lengthening it. Rest on one side of the back, arms on one side, and legs relaxed.

- Supta Padangusthasana-(Big Toe Pose)-
  relieves back pain, stretches knees, hamstrings,
  and opens the lower back to allow the energy
  from the kidneys, the meridians of the bladder
  to flow in.

Lie on the stomach, raise the shoulder with one hip,
and the leg stays straight with the foot flexed. Place
the harness around the leg ball and straighten it out.
Hold your back loose, and your arms straight and
nose gently close to the chest. Keep and relax, as the
bowels and hamstring. Press the tail to the ground as
exhaled and stretch forward with both thighs. The
raised leg doesn't have to be upright, just straight.
Keep a few breaths and then switch hands.

- Paripurna Navasana (Boat Pose) — covers the
  lower back of the kidneys and abdominals.
  Hold your feet on the ground, or hug your legs
  while you stabilize and push on.

Lie down on your chest buttocks and cover your legs.
Continue to align your bones and raise your feet off
the surface, feeling the belly involved. Raise your
footsteps slowly parallel to the floor, bend your knees,
lean back 30-40 degrees and raise your arms, touch
your knees and parallel to the floor. Continue to relax,
work the mulabhanda, and bring all your energy to
your center. After a few steps, Hold knees to the chest.

- Virasana (Seated Hero Pose)-Meditate to complete the workout. Excellent for emotional relaxation and intestinal fire centering. Concentrate on Mulabhanda painting. An alternative for mediation is Savasana (Corpse Pose).

Lay your back, long legs, side-arms, and head with the blanket if necessary. The rolling pillow under the legs with an eye bag or shielding the head. Fully relax and concentrate on your body, release all limbs, bones, organs, and skin to the earth in harmony and abandonment. Last at least 5 minutes, and then roll up and curl into a ball before you finish.

Practice every day, and it will take 20 minutes, slowly grow up by keeping poses for more breaths and taking care of your life, how you feed yourself, and how you want to live. Can expand to a range of expression without intense pain.

The safest way to meditate is on a leaky butt, and ideally at sunrise or sunset after your asanas.

In short, it is not shocking that some of the highest figures for prostate (and breast) cancers are found in the North. Why? For me, we could place too much attention on the body and related material paraphernalia, while we might concentrate not only on our own Soul and abilities but also on each other. Perhaps if we turned back our minds, started to live in a pleasant way more frequently, ceased to experience and enjoy the world below our feet, which gives us what we need, these numbers may be diminished and supplemented with high self-esteem, resilience and constant joy! Are we bold enough to envision such a planet, let alone build it?

It all starts with us as individuals, so yoga is so powerful. We are all the same in our beds, we all have the same muscles, we feel the same feelings, and we acknowledge our shortcomings and successes in our friend. Yoga helps us hear, relax, and take care of it. It lets us laugh at ourselves (which we're not doing enough of) and enflames our emotional and caring existence. And the kind of force that burns inside you will make it impossible for you to remain alight.

Traditional therapy-When you don't believe you have a prostate problem, it's necessary to get it checked out by the Doctor. Traditional care. Digital rectal (DRE) scans or urinary, and blood testing can determine whether or not you have Benign Prostate Hyperplasia or other prostate disorders, so a prostate cancer screening check will be performed.

Frequently Asked Yoga Questions

Yoga is a perfect workout if you want to take form and cope with pain. It's a habit everyone will continue for the remainder of their lives. If you intend to take yoga, read, and find answers to some of the questions you often pose.

If I'm not very strong, can I even do yoga? Yoga isn't all about endurance, sure you can. It's about relaxing and poses. You will realize through yoga that you are always getting more versatile, please don't drive yourself too hard. Space is required.

Do men practice yoga? Do they do? Yeah, of course. Yeah, of course. Yoga has recently been even more famous among men in recent years. Men all enjoy the same advantages as women, such as increased resilience, strength, and decreased tension.

How did yoga come from, and when? Yoga has been in India for thousands and thousands of years. There will be anything about it because it has suffered this for many years.

Is yoga going to help me lose weight? Yes, yoga can assist you in weight loss. It gives you the discipline to maintain a healthy lifestyle, to eliminate junk food temptations, and to relieve stress. Stress causes you to gain weight and may reduce your weight.

How frequently should I do yoga? A good start would be to go twice a week for a 60-minute course. It is hard, however, to overdo it, and you would be in good shape if you could do 30 minutes each day. Every day, a little bit is better at once.

Hope your questions on yoga have been answered in this book. You can contact a nearby Yoga Studio in your area if you need more information. Take one or two courses, and you're not going to be disappointed.

YOGA FOR PREGNANT WOMEN

Pregnancy is a daunting event; it constitutes one of the most critical times in women's lives and is thus regarded often with much concern by most women. It is because of this that pregnant women influenced by the experience of yoga highly suggest this type of physics to many women who are generally at the crossroads and uncertain about their shifts. However, sound sense maintains that, before embarkation, all new processes and their approaches must first be researched carefully, and that is also applicable to yoga for pregnant women.

Since it is a new idea, there will naturally be specific questions the women will pose about the course, and some of the problems sometimes asked about it are discussed as follows: Why is yoga so different for pregnant women? Yoga is considered unique for expectant mothers since, aside from giving the intended mother the requisite amount of physical exercise during this time, it also contributes to spiritual and emotional strengthening. A widespread assumption during the pregnancy is that the baby's mental status depends on the mother's health, and thus if she is healthy and well adjusted, happy, and stress-free, there are strong chances that the baby will be the same.

Will it be healthy as a workout during pregnancy? Sure, if yoga is carried out under the expertise of a skilled practitioner who understands the specific circumstances of breastfeeding, it is not only healthy but ideal for pregnant women.

Will it affect the planned mother abstractly? Yoga is based on the concepts of wisdom and self-awareness development that are accomplished by meditation and guided breathing exercises. Training in these areas during pregnancy would also not only ensure the mother's stable mental health but also make a significant contribution to the small life within it.

How long will one stop exercising before delivery? Yoga is preferably designed to work for pregnant women during the three trimesters, but that depends solely on particular conditions in the sense that if the nursing woman feels upset, it will interrupt the practice and follow the advice of the doctor.

What can potential wellness benefits for pregnant women be achieved by yoga? Including physical health over the whole cycle of breastfeeding, there are a variety of other lifetime advantages which can be obtained by yoga for pregnant mothers, with the most significant being the elimination of the extra flab and the ugly stretch marks.

CONCLUSION

Many people are actively seeking to better their health and sometimes search for new ways of achieving so. Dieting is a fad of the past and also general fitness with new methods claiming to remove weight and sound muscle. Yoga is one of the latest ways to build the body. Not to suggest that you don't need a balanced diet, but in combination with daily yoga instruction, you would be shocked by the results. Yet yoga is also not only about physical fitness, and the effects go way beyond the physical aspect.

Because of the physical benefits that are so important to you from yoga, we will discuss them first. Yoga helps us to teach ourselves to claim the right pose regardless of what we do. The specific poses aid not only to relax our body's muscles but also to exercise them. Yoga also allows blood to circulate by breathing exercises that help the body obtain the required amount of oxygen. Everything that allows the brain to function correctly. While we don't really speak about these facets about good wellbeing, changing these things will definitely make a difference in the way we act.

The second most significant benefit you'll learn from yoga is the subconscious. Yoga is an ideal way to calm the mind and reduce everyday stress. The methods used, including the poses and breathing, are intended to relax the mind and soul and allow us to release toxic energy. Practicing yoga can also allow you to properly integrate your mind and body. It alone will be raising discomfort both in the body and in spirit, tremendously. That gives one a happier feeling.

Yoga also has other wellness benefits. Weight management and physical changes help to enhance our mental wellbeing. A balanced body and mind contribute to a robust immune system that enables you to fight illness and infection. Yoga helps you retain your usual weight, increase your physical strength, boost your memory and alertness, and even leave your body feeling healthy throughout the exercise. The general sense of health will become a regular feature of your life soon after you learn to practice yoga.

It is a significant choice to take over your life and to stick to some schedule. Individuals should contact a practitioner before every diet or workout regimen begins. Yoga is a relatively healthy exercise, but those who have controlled issues can have to consider ways to support themselves to maintain their physical health. You will want to buy a relaxing mat during your workout before starting, and you may want to find a sweet spot to work in. You will quickly discover the many effects of yoga and perform much healthier than ever before. Most people are actively seeking to change their health, and many people are looking for new ways to do so. Dieting is a fad of the past and also general fitness with new methods claiming to remove weight and sound muscle. Yoga is one of the latest ways to build the body. Not to suggest that you don't need a balanced diet, but in combination with daily yoga instruction, you would be shocked by the results. Yet yoga is also not only about physical fitness, and the effects go way beyond the physical aspect.

Because of the physical benefits that are so important to you from yoga, we will discuss them first. Yoga helps us to teach ourselves to claim the right pose regardless of what we do. The specific poses aid not only to relax our body's muscles but also to exercise them. Yoga also allows blood to circulate by breathing exercises that help the body obtain the required amount of oxygen. Everything that allows the brain to function correctly. While we don't really speak about these facets about good wellbeing, changing these things will definitely make a difference in the way we act.

The second most significant benefit you'll learn from yoga is the subconscious. Yoga is an ideal way to calm the mind and reduce everyday stress. The methods used, including the poses and breathing, are intended to relax the mind and soul and allow us to release toxic energy. Practicing yoga can also allow you to properly integrate your mind and body. It alone will be raising discomfort both in the body and in spirit, tremendously. That gives one a happier feeling.

Yoga also has other wellness benefits. Weight management and physical changes help to enhance our mental wellbeing. A balanced body and mind contribute to a robust immune system that enables you to fight illness and infection. Yoga helps you retain your usual weight, increase your physical strength, boost your memory and alertness, and even leave your body feeling healthy throughout the exercise. The general sense of health will become a regular feature of your life soon after you learn to practice yoga.

It is a significant choice to take over your life and to stick to some schedule. Individuals should contact a practitioner before every diet or workout regimen begins. Yoga is a relatively healthy exercise, but those who have controlled issues can have to consider ways to support themselves to maintain their physical health. You will want to buy a relaxing mat during your workout before starting, and you may want to find a sweet spot to work in. Within the near future, you will learn the many advantages of yoga, and probably you feel better than ever.